TOSHIBA

Beyond Vitruvius

A Unified View Of Strength and The Fundamental Properties of the Universe

James Baird

10/31/2013

Beyond Vitruvius

A Unified View of Strength and the Fundamental Properties of the Universe

Copyright ©2013

By James Baird

DISCLAIMER : The information in this book is presented in good faith, but no warranty is given, or results guaranteed. None of the information contained in this book is intended to be taken as medical advice. Consult a physician before engaging in any strenuous exercise program. The author and publisher are not responsible for any injury, damage, losses, claims, actions, procedures or expenses that result from using the advice or instructions in this book.

This book is dedicated to Laura Bur, Betty and Pudge – for their help and indulgence

A quick introduction

The westerner views man and motion as two separate things that can be described in terms of artistic value (physical "beauty") or mathematical formulae. Both of these approaches only measure the *appearances* of underlying functions. Measuring and judging the quality of every nose on earth will not tell you how a nose works or what, exactly, is the sensation of "smell".

Everything in the universe arises from only 92 (or so) elements, and everything on Earth is basically made of only *four* of these elements. And every element arises from a singularity – an unknowable something (or no-thingness). At that point of singularity, there is nothing to measure – any measurement comes *after* the generative function.

That is what this book is about – the functions that underlie human motion *before* the application of tags and labels and measures. I tried to make simple some very complex ideas and perhaps went too far with gross oversimplification. But my intention is to make science something understandable and, above all, *useable*.

There is the universe. The word "universe" is simply a label. What we experience as the universe has other labels – the tao, the zero point field, the void, the unknowable, etc.

The universe has different forms, but they are not separate from the universe. Everything in the universe is *of* the universe. And any changes that take place are changes in form only. The "stuff" of the universe doesn't change; it can neither be created nor destroyed. It can only change form.

People became very excited when they realized that light has a "dual nature" and can appear as both particle (solid form) and wave (energy form). This is somewhat misleading because it implies that light is separate from the universe. That light can have more than one form is obvious if you consider that light is a form of the universe and the universe possesses all forms.

So we next have to understand that the words particle, wave, solid, and energy are descriptive labels applied to distinctive phases of a single universe.

In a way, these words seem redundant. But they are necessary tools for communicating experiences and concepts. We just have to be careful to remember that " distinct" does not mean *different*.

To describe anything that happens is to describe the universe happening. There is not a universe and then a separate "you" doing stuff. That you move "in accordance with the universe" sounds all mystical and eastern and is a difficult concept for most westerners to accept. So I'm going to try to make my point by using baseball as an illustrative tool.

Visualize the entire playing field as different points about the size of a baseball. If I hit a fly ball to a point in left field and it takes three seconds to reach that point, the path of the ball will describe an arc. If I hit a ball to that same point so that it only takes two seconds to get there, the ball's path will have a different arc. I can't make the ball arrive in two seconds with a "three second arc".

A ball hit to any point and the time it takes to get there will have a specific arc that it will share with no other hit. You can't impose your will on the ball and make it do anything you want. The ball moves in accordance with the universe.

This time-space structure is why the earth follows an elliptical path around the sun. The earth isn't falling toward the sun — the earth is moving in a straight path; it is spacetime that curves. Another way of looking at this is to imagine drawing a straight line on a piece of paper. The line is straight but can be curved by curving the paper.

To describe human movement is to describe macrocosmic activities in a microcosmic form. Remember: you can't do anything that is contrary to how the universe does anything. The key to improving your performance (and health in general) is realizing and accepting this.

To begin with, we have to understand some terms. Everything is some form of the universe, but there are some distinctions. These distinctions are not "things" unto themselves, but are qualities being expressed. We want to grow away from overly simplified labeling and see that if everything is a form of one thing, then any qualities being expressed are transitory and relative.

Solid, for instance, describes something having dimensions that are uniform and coherently associated. Solidity is a quality that resists fluid deformation and retains it's structural integrity. So we can accurately describe timespace as solid or expressing solid qualities.

Energy or energetic describes something dynamically transitive. It is fluid, freely associative, but not necessarily unstable. The thing about energy is that it requires a dimensional medium –a solid form- in order to manifest. There is no energy without dimension or a solid quality. There is energy commited to a specific form and a fluid form of energy, but there is structure in that fluidity.

Waves are an example of this. Waves are variances that transfer energy progressively from one point to another. This variance can be in the form of elastic deformation or gradients in pressure or intensity. The term I prefer to use for all this is angular modulation.

Waves occur in different forms and in a variety of mediums. In a bullwhip, the angular modulation appears in the sine wave form that travels along the length of rawhide. Waves in jell-o appear as oscillating angles. In a toy Slinky, each coil only slightly adjusts its position as the wave energy passes through. The point is that the wave doesn't require the "wavy" appearance of the ocean surf. Energy infuses a medium and the medium exhibits a particular "wavy" quality.

Let's look at waves a little differently. Waves don't have to move. Any information can be converted to wave form and then transformed back (sometimes called Fourier transforms). Sound waves can be converted and stored as binary codes in a computer or as magnetic patterns on a tape. They can even be converted to musical notations and represented on paper and then transformed back into music. So the sound waves went from a fluid form to a distinctively solid form and them back to fluid.

In your ears, sound waves transform into mechanical pressure waves and then into electric waves. But there is also speakers and amplifiers and instruments and singers all making waves and all of these waves undergo continual transformations.

On a tighter scale, we have atoms. Atoms are often thought of as particles or being made of particles. But really an atom is a local system of transformations. There is fluid energy (atomic forces) organizing and expressing less-fluid properties (protons and neutrons) that organize a semi-solid quality (the electron cloud). Atoms are simply a very localized microcosmic expression of transformations; much like a single piece of music can undergo a series of conversions and still represent the same information – no notes are lost in the transition between a recording and your ear.

All this talk of transformations and atoms and whatnot is not just page filler. There are grand implications here and they don't simply *concern* your movement; they ARE your movements. So bear with me a bit while I hammer away at certain points.

Spacetime is a symmetrically structured , solid form of the universe. And ALL transformations and movements are fluidly symmetrical forms of spacetime. A grossly oversimplified comparison can be made with a chess board.The symmetry of the checkerboard pattern defines and shapes the game as a whole. Every move is governed by, and is an expression of, the relationship between the pieces and the board. Chess is both fluid in its expression and solid in its coherent structure. The labels "fluid" and "solid" describe the same event.

Now, let's return to music as an illustrative tool. Music is simply a coherent structure of sound waves. A specific song exhibits even greater uniformity. The archetypal idea of music is a fluid concept. Your favorite song is a concrete idea – it is solid in nature; you can't change its structure or it no longer represents your favorite tune. You can, however, alter its format. It can exist on your i-phone, or on a c.d. or you can hear it on the radio or television, etc. So we can see that solid and fluid aren't as different as they appear to be; they are labels used to distinguish between phase states of a singularity. And this singularity (in the case of music) is the angular modulation of molecules. No angular modulation in a medium – no sounds. All the solid/ fluid dynamics and transformations of sound/music are expressions of a single function.

Before we can go forward to movement and strength, we have to go back – all the way to the "big bang". Before the cosmos came into being, there was just the unknowable. It wasn't unknowable because it was so mysterious, it was simply indistinct. It was undifferentiated. The universe didn't come from "nothing" so much as no thing- no distinct thing.

Imagine there was nothing but flatness. No dimensions. And just grey. No shades, just grey. You wouldn't even be aware of greyness or flatness. Because there would be no distinctions. You would be surrounded by grey and flat (you would even be grey and flat) and you would never know it. There would be no "you" to even be grey and flat. This is a glimpse into unknowability. There is something, but no way to know about it.

So, in the beginning, there was undifferentiated potential. Then distinction occurs. This kick-off could have been the "big bang", but not necessarily. The "big bang" itself could be reflective of other underlying processes.

From the sudden expansion, the universe expresses distinct forms. It's important to keep in mind that these are distinctive forms of one thing and not separate things unto themselves. The first forms were simple distinctions- fluid timespace in a solid timespace structure or, waves of energy. All kinds of wave forms- light waves, radio waves, heat, and so on. And again, not different- just distinct.

For example, the sun compresses hydrogen into helium and this process releases energy that takes the forms of heat, light, color, electromagnetism- radiation of all kinds. One process – many forms. The same laser light you experience as the color red can also be experienced as heat on your skin.

We now come to the **big revelation.** All processes and distinctions are based on **angular modulation.**

Every molecule, every atom, every variance in tension and compression are all based on an angular relationships. Every change happens through angular modulation, but angulation is not the *cause* of change. Change and angulation are flip sides of the same coin. Change, distinction and angulation are inseparable, as is the energy released or absorbed during angular changes.

Solid is a slower angular change while "energy" is a more rapid angular adjustment. It all has to be as simple as angular modulation because **it's all one thing**. Think about it. In the beginning, there was one undifferentiated potential . And everything since is still simply a form of that one thing.

For instance, let's say that you put your hands under the sheets on your bed to form different shapes (maybe you're playing with your pet cat). The bedsheet is one undifferentiated field and the only distinctions arise from the different angles you make with your hands.

Spacetime is the bedsheet and the angulations of the sheet would be areas of pressure variances like stars and galaxies. And where these pressure variances occur, different threads in the spacetime bedsheet would become apparent. The different threads are the 92 basic elements that are found throughout the timespace continuum. These elements are not different from the spacetime stuff; they are an apparent *form* of spacetime stuff.

The thing to take from all this is that there is only conversion of energy. Conservation of energy is only conversion at a slower rate.

Your physical structure represents a form of stored energy. The energy you store is generated by the relationship of the angular momentum of earth and the spacetime substance. There is no "gravity" that pulls on you like a magnet. Imagine that you are deep in the ocean and a submarine comes along and runs into you. Now, it's propelling you along at a speed fast enough that you are plastered to the submarine and the force of the water is pulling at your mask and fins and breathing equipment. You wouldn't think that what you are experiencing is due to some mysterious, magnetic force pulling you to the submarine.

But this is similar to the experience we have on earth; The earth accelerates us while there is also tremendous atmospheric pressure being exerted at the same time. The atmosphere itself exerts thousands of pounds of pressure on you constantly. So when you jump into the air, the earth accelerates into you while the air pushes into you with the crushing pressure of an ocean. There is no magnetic, pulling force needed.

When you lift a weight, the term "lift weight" is not entirely accurate. It's a simple term and is suitable for conversational use. But if you want to understand how you really work, we have to be far more precise. You and the weight both have a specific angular relationship to earth. You alter your angular relationship (your structure) and you transfer the energy generated by your changing relationship into the weight, whose change in angular relationship to the earth is marked by a curved path.

But this event is not actually a separate "you" acting on an object. Once you connect with the weight, you form a single unit. It would be a little different if you were running up to the weight and kicking it to generate acceleration, but when you take hold of a weight, its energetic relationship to earth now joins with yours.

Let's go back to the baseball illustration where energy transformation is a little easier to see. When you throw a baseball, your wind up is a series of fluid angular changes. These changes generate energy that you then release. The ball's flight expresses the energy that you generated. The ball is literally representing a pulse of energy. You can observe this delivery of energy when you see a person break a stack of bricks with a punch. When the strike is delivered, a wave of energy travels through the bricks with enough force to break the bonded structure of multiple bricks, even though the strike only made contact with the surface of one brick.

When the baseball is hit by a bat, there is a combining of forces and this energetic exchange is represented by the curved path of the ball. What is important to see is that the thrown ball, the swung bat and the ball's path after being hit are not discrete events. The pitcher and the batter both transformed energy (friction, earth's acceleration and bioenergy) and the path of the ball was a visible form of that energy conversion.

There were other forms of that energetic conversion: the ball and bat deformed at the moment of impact and vibrations ran down the length of the bat. There was energy released as sound (the crack of the bat) and there was a bit of heat generated as well.

From baseball, I want to explore a macro example of the how fluidly energy can express the same thing in multiple forms. A star can be considered as an angulation of spacetime. This angular activity generates enough energy (in the form of pressure) to convert Hydrogen into Helium. This conversion is accompanied by a release of heat and light. As a star goes through energetic changes, increases in heat and pressure convert Helium into Carbon, then Oxygen, Nitrogen, Magnesium and so on. And every conversion is represented by a specific wavelength of energy that we observe as color. So each change in the star's behavior is recorded by a wavelength of light, a specific atomic structure (shape) with particular chemical properties as well as sound and other forms of radiation.

Each element formed expresses a specific color so that you could look at a spectrum of color given off by a star and determine what elements are present. Here's the thing: each and every expression of the same stellar activity will have **a specific angular signature.** No matter how many forms of the same event there are, they can all be seen as angular representations of a greater angular modulation. If it can be said that there is a single, primary form of information in the universe, it is angulation.

When you ball up a piece of paper, that crumpled appearance is an angular representation of the energy you applied. The wrinkled hood of a car that has been in an accident captures the wave of energy generated in the collision. These wave patterns are recorded information.

In the above examples, waves are seen as a way of capturing information about an event. When waves interact and form an interference pattern (similar to what you see when you drop multiple objects into a pool of water), a surprising amount of information is generated and stored.

An illustration of the unbelievable amount of information generated by multiple waves interacting is holographic photography. A hologram is a three dimensional image of an object created by splitting a beam of laser light and bouncing one of the beams off the object being photographed. The two beams are then reunited on a piece of holographic film. When the two beams combine, an interference pattern is recorded. Now when a laser beam is passed through the film, a three dimensional image of the photographed object appears.

Interestingly, if you cut the film into small pieces, each piece will reproduce the whole three dimensional image. You can also capture multiple images on a single piece of film by adjusting the angle at which the laser beams act on the film.

The reason for these long explanations of energy conversion and timespace structure and atomic activity is that people today (westerners in particular) are quick to dismiss the roles that energy conversion and universal structure play in our daily lives. It is disturbingly common for people to behave as if they were some isolated brain-entity locked in a mechanical transport system navigating along on some alien planet. This viewpoint represents an almost psychotic break from reality.

But because this is such a deeply ingrained belief system, I am forced to go back to the creation of the universe and work my way through every detail of existence in order to show that the true power available in the universe lies in its symmetry. It does no good to struggle to impose your will on the universe because you are not separate from the universe. The only way for you to make changes is to understand how the universe makes transformations. There is no other way.

While I'm on the subject of stupid beliefs that exhibit remarkable longevity, **your limbs do not act as levers.** We've all been subjected to the image of the bicep and forearm working as a lever. First and foremost, your muscles don't pull (or contract) like a cable of some kind. Your muscles don't directly connect to any bones anywhere. And your muscles don't connect directly to each other (not even between the fibers).

I want to point out that the lever(and every other of the basic simple machines – inclined plane, pulley, wheel and axle, and screw) is an expression of angular modulation. By changing angles, you express a conversion of time and space, generating energy transformation. We call this transformation "work" and we define work as force times distance applied (in the same direction). Levers are basically distance amplifiers. When you use pliers or turn a door handle (or knob), these devices allow you to apply force over a greater distance and longer time on a central point.

The problem with defining the arm as a lever is that it only looks like a lever; it does not operate like one except in the broadest sense of an energy converter.

The biggest reason that you cannot consider the human body as a collection of levers and simple machinery is that the human being is a complex, nonlinear system of functions that display emergent characteristics.

Before we continue, you need to have some grasp of how different systems operate. We'll start with linear systems. A linear system is comprised of linear functions. The term "function" simply refers to a relationship between one thing and another. The function of glue is to bond surfaces together. The bonding function is considered linear because its purpose doesn't change even if the types of surface material varies. In math, addition would be a linear function because addition works the same way no matter what numbers are being plugged in. A lever, of course, is a linear function.

A kite can represent a linear *system*. A kite is composed of components whose functions are invariate. The sticks, paper, tail and line each have a specific purpose and are not interchangeable. One of the hallmarks of a linear system is that you can take it apart and reassemble it and the pieces always add up – they always do the same things in the same way.

Nonlinear behavior is much more difficult to define. Basically, nonlinear describes the behavior of a system that cannot be obtained (or explained) by the summing of its constituent parts. But it's so much more than that. Grasping nonlinearity is a major step towards understanding and improving your physical abilities.

Say that a linear equation was composed of two mechanical systems interacting (This is an excellent example because this is how most "trainers" and "experts" see the body). In this equation, as interaction between the systems increased or decreased, the behavior of each system would alter in a predictable manner- if there was a small increase in interaction, then the behavior of each system would change by a correspondingly small amount. If the interaction was zero, the mechanical behavior would be that of two independent systems. So small changes result in small effects.

A nonlinear equation/system cannot be solved or added together. In a nonlinear equation of two interacting mechanical systems, as interaction increases or decreases, the behavior of the systems might change slowly and predictably as a parameter is reached and then suddenly **BAM**! There's a change to a totally new behavior. And this change will be dramatic, unpredictable and disproportionate. A whole range of values or conditions will reflect in behavior that is regular and predictable but some infinitesimal variance will throw the entire system into a wholly new state.

A concept similar to nonlinearity is emergence. Emergence is sometimes called *synergy* and basically indicates much coming from little. In other words, the outcome is much greater than the sum of the parts would indicate. How does this differ from nonlinearity? Nonlinearity has a chaotic element to it.

I'll use driving a car as an illustration. The gas and brake are simple functions and comprise a linear system- there is a predictable correspondence between their interactions and small changes equal small effects. When you add in steering, the system becomes a little more complex; each function has a direct effect on the other functions and their interactions together are a little different than their individual behavior. The first step into nonlinearity comes in the form of friction. Friction expresses the amount of energy needed for steering, acceleration and deceleration. But the amount of energy changes depending on how fast you are going, the angle and condition of you tires, road conditions, etc. When you factor in other drivers and all of the strange and stupid behavior that people exhibit while behind the wheel, you can easily see how driving suddenly went from a nice, simple mechanical interaction to a system of chaos.

A school of fish exemplifies emergent behavior. A school of fish displays all sorts of intricate movement patterns and shape changes while still maintaining a coherent association. And all this complex activity couldn't be predicted by studying the behavior of one or two fish.

The school of fish also illustrates what could be called leadership from the "bottom up". Simply, there is no single "lead" fish. There is no select group of fish that assesses changing conditions and issues appropriate orders to be executed. Rather, the complex group behavior arises from everyone following a few simple rules, such as " swim with fish similar to you but don't bump into anyone" and "if two or more of your neighbors turn, turn with them". And from these simple rules arises surprisingly complex patterns of activity.

So, an emergent system is one in which a small number of interactions generates behaviors of surprising complexity, while still maintaining recognizable and recurring features. The complexity will not be random in nature and will be regular, if not predictable.

Nonlinearity will definitely display a random quality and the arising behavior may bear no apparent resemblance to the initial states.

Non-mechanical equations, such as human behavior, can display several different operating systems at the same time. If you observe children on a playground, their interactions will be based on simple natural rules (stick with those that are familiar; if a group seems to be having fun, follow their lead), top down instruction (behaving as they were taught by parents) and a random, nonlinear element (you can't predict who will get along with whom or for how long).

I mentioned bottom-up behavior systems, where interactions at a lower level without a central control determines the actions of the system as a whole. The polar opposite of this type of system is a top- down hierarchy. In this form of organization, there is a central control that directs the activities of the entire system.

Originally, this was the approach to computer programming. Programmers tried to write rules and specific responses to cover every situation. But the computer could not deal with random variances because its programmed behavior was too inflexible. The computer would make mistakes. New rules were added to avoid those mistakes, which led to different mistakes and more rules and so on. The programs quickly grew to gigantic proportions with millions of lines of code. Then, the programs would fail out of sheer complexity. Programmers could no longer figure out where the mistakes were being generated. Unfortunately, the top- down hierarchy is still the model being used to explain how the brain controls movement.

Computer programming today is based on examples from nature. The new method involves the use of a **distributed network.** This network is made up of many agents with only basic level interactions obeying simple rules. The behavior of the system as a whole is NOT pre-programmed, but instead arises from the interactions of the agents in the network.

The failure of the top- down system is that it restricts or eliminates free interactions at the initial levels. To see why unrestricted lower level interactions are so important, I'll use ants as an example. An ant colony operates as a distributed network also, where the state of the colony as a whole is determined by the outcome of basic interactions among the general population.

Ants self- organize according to changing needs and conditions. And these needs are defined by the number of interactions an ant has. If an ant encounters lots of foraging ants, then it will find another need to fulfill; perhaps it will work on mound building or go on trash duty. The ant can only accurately assess needs by a high number of contacts. Only seeing three ants will not provide insight into the general state of the colony compared to coming across hundreds of ants.

The strength of this sort of operational system is that the nonlinearity of widespread interactions allows for fluid responses to changing conditions and uncertainty without dependence on rigid orders from a high command.

There is yet another type of organizing system that we have to discuss. This is not so much a system as it is an emergent behavior of a system. It works by **resonance.** A resonant system begins as a bottom- up type of organization. Certain patterns arise from lower level interactions that start to influence the behavior of the overall system. But at some point, the influencing patterns take on a life of their own and begin to dictate the actions of the lower level agents. The behavior of the lower agents now reinforces the dictating patterns, which in turn alters the distributed network even more.

A perfect example of this phenomenon is money. At some point, some people decided to assign a corresponding symbolic value to unrelated items, like one goat will be worth ten chickens; or a pound of copper and two pounds of tin will be of equal value to two bolts of cloth and one shiny stone and so on. But somewhere along the way, symbolic wealth started to determine the value of the people who created the concept to begin with. Now, symbolic wealth (money) has taken on the mantle of a powerful organizing force. Money decides which people live or die, where and how will live, the quality of education, etc.

Money now organizes and dictates the behavior of people globally even though the existence of money is not intrinsic to survival. There are still cultures that operate by the barter system or by a system of pooled resources.

The power of resonance is such that ANY form of organization that resonates can exhibit a synergistic behavior that unfolds in unbelievably complex and powerful ways – even greater than nonlinearity would indicate.

In an emergent, nonlinear system, it's impossible to use observations and measurements of the beginning state to predict the mature form. And you cannot use observations of the mature form to predict the structure of the beginning state.

I'll use a birthday cake as an example. If you were to look at the ingredients separately (the sugar,the salt ,flour, eggs,etc.), you would not be able to predict the appearance of the finished product. And studying the finished product does not allow you to predict the component elements or the emergent process that took place. If you didn't know what a cake was, you could eat all the cake you want and never divine the process or ingredients that went into the cake.

In a resonant system, the beginning state and the mature form influence each other to such an extent that there is no longer any way to separate the two and any distinctions are relative and arbitrary. Organic life on earth is an example of this. Marked by restless and perpetual shifts in behavior, every plant, animal and insect changes in response to the activity of every other plant, animal and insect with every passing instant. Biological systems are so complex that you cannot know in advance the eventual consequences of anything you do.

The act of resonant organization can transform the immaterial into material form. The concept of symbolic wealth – the idea of money - is strictly immaterial. It has no inherent physical form. Most of the people who use money don't understand it and even fear it. Yet, it has generated not only a palpable existence, but has developed concrete forms such as the buildings that house banking and lending businesses and institutions for financial speculation .

Resonant organization can be used to describe the transformation of quarks into particles, molecules into amino acids and amino acids into proteins , cells and organs.

Top- down organization is always an emergent property, since no system just pops into existence, fully formed and possessing a complete working knowledge of the universe. Even though the lever is a simple machine, it's still an organized system that is not inherent to the universe. So, humans cannot be made of levers any more than cars can just grow on trees.

Everything in the universe has to go through a developmental phase that is inseparable from the mature form.

For example, a herd of cattle can be cloned from a single egg and raised together in the same environment. Yet, the individual cows will develop distinct personality traits and behavior patterns and these distinctions will lead to internal changes even though the outer appearances are identical.

Most people don't realize that DNA is not fixed. You are NOT born with a complete set of blueprints that determines the parameters of your life. This sort of hierarchy would constitute a strictly top- down system that is not in line with reality. DNA interacts with your daily activities and environment and changes over time.

Genes have insulators and promoters that manipulate genetic activity by isolating specific sequences or acting as switches that turn sections on or off. A single gene sequence can code for multiple proteins while other sections are only activated by environmental factors or the actions of some other genetic sequence.

There are even human chimeras- people that possess two different sets of DNA. Their skin might contain one kind of DNA strand while their kidney will have another.

Like DNA, people too often consider the brain to be some omniscient controller of all human activity. But the brain does not represent, nor does it have access to, some universal schematic or instructional almanac.

A healthy brain itself functions just fine; it's the usage of the brain and the emergent production that is so often inappropriate, misguided or just plain wrong.

The brain, like movement itself, is a complex, nonlinear system. Actually, there is NO separation between brain and movement; they both have component elements, but together make one distributed network that displays a resonant organization.

For example, how would the hand and its function be differentiated? Do you say that the hand only extends from fingertips to the wrist? The muscles and tendons that generate hand activity are mainly in the forearm. And the forearm's function is inseparable from the upper arm which is reflective of the activities of the pectorals and the deltoids and so on and so forth.

And any of the actions taken by the physical components are highly dependent on neurological input (and vice versa). Much of the brain's area is dedicated to the mapping of specific physical functions. This mapping is disproportionately represented by the hands, feet, face, lips and genitals with hands, feet and lips being primarily depicted. If you were to construct a little doll based on the proportions mapped by the brain, it would resemble a sort of "Mr. Potato Head" with monstrously huge lips, hands and feet on a tiny torso with teeny little arms and legs.

So, you can see that pinning down the exact location and function of the hand is not as simple as you might first think.

Both the brain and movement systems (if considered separately) work in a holographic manner. There are many weak, asymmetrical links (as opposed to a few strong, linear connections controlling the rest of the system). Each of these links generates waves of information that unite and create interference patterns. The distributed weak links act as multiple agents, allowing small deviations to cascade into large effects. The system of weak linkages and waves of activity encourages wholistic activity that can respond robustly to any situational changes.

With a widely distributed network of loose associations, a solitary signal has little chance of reaching some distant point to which there is no direct or linear connection. But a group of spiking electric activity firing together (if not simultaneously) and propogating in waves carries much more informational power than even a similarly sized spiking group activating in a less unified form.

Similar to DNA, there is no set sequence that acts autonomously on the system as a whole. For instance, the only time you have a "knee" or "back" or "foot" is in describing a point of disfunction or acute injury. In a healthy system, the behavior of these anatomical distinctions are highly dependent on the activities of other functions- even those that are not close by or directly connected. In other words, a back or knee problem is more likely an issue of angulation among distributed points.

One of the greatest advantages of a widely distributed network of many agents is the ability to detect patterns, even when those patterns are in a very subtle form. The strength of this advantage is dependent upon a high number of interactions (like the self-organization of ant colonies).

Another illustration of the "wisdom of the masses" effect happened when a cow was being offered as a prize at some rural state fair. The winning contestant was to be the person who could guess the weight of the cow. When all of the guesses were recorded and compared, no one had won. But it was later discovered that if all of the guesses were added together and averaged, the result turned out to be correct within a few decimal points!

This phenomenon was studied using various guessing games (like how many jelly beans or pennies a huge jar contained). The effect occurred time and time again. No one person had the correct information, but somehow, a large group of people exhibited a "combined wisdom".

Neuroanatomy implies that the brain operates from clearly delineated compartments. But like your body's anatomy, these distinctions are not to be confused with the workings of the system as a whole. After all, if you dismantled your television, you would find a high degree of organized compartmentalization; you could easily separate the components that regulate color, sound, volume, color, graphics, and so on.

But none of these mechanisms is the originator of the information that they regulate. The components are transformers and mediators of information, rather than *controllers* of information.

Your clock is an expression of time, but the clock doesn't control time, nor do the component parts *contain* time. Just as your television is a tool for broadcasting, but is not the broadcasting itself.

If you can grasp this concept, you can then see why you (and your brain) are very often easily misled by people or by misreading a situation. This is why you have to *learn* how to walk and talk and do anything and everything else and why everyone expresses (and experiences) things differently and why we often respond inappropriately to situations. **It's because there is no one part of you that is in control , nor is there a single correct response to anything**. Your brain is part of a global system that converts, interprets, stores and extrapolates information.

Your brain does not "make sense" out of a disordered mass of sensory input. The input you sense already has an ordered structure even before it reaches you. For example, when you smell some "thing", you are actually responding to the geometry (shape) of a molecule.

When you experience hearing, it is a response to logarithmic, proportional differences in frequencies. And logarithmic expansion is a geometric expression of spirals.

Vision is conversion of electromagnetic (light) waves and touch is sensitivity to vibration.

Much of the time, our sensory input is undifferentiated until our brains start making distinctions and associations, but undifferentiated doesn't mean disordered. An unopened box of crayons is an undifferentiated whole until you open it up and start combining and associating the colors you find inside (draw and color). But that doesn't mean that the crayons were some crazy, random mass of information before you started making your drawing. Your artwork is an expression of an order that *you* impose.

Here are some examples of a hidden order for you to consider.

If you pluck a guitar string, a note sounds. If you then press the string at its halfway point and sound that note, you get the same note, but twice as high as the first. The vibrational frequency has a 2:1 ratio.

A hammer weighing half as much as another will strike a note twice as high. Again, a 2:1 expression. All simple instruments behave the same way, whether plucked, struck or blown.

Pendulums of equal length will always take the same amount of time to execute one swing – regardless of weight, force applied or geometry of arc; pendulum length , time and distance of swing are inseparable.

Now, a harmonograph is a device comprised of two (or sometimes three) pendulums suspended through holes in a table that swing at angles to each other. Above the table, the shaft of one pendulum carries an arm with a pen and the other pendulum shaft carries a platform with a piece of paper attached to it. As the pendulums swing, the result of their combined motion makes a drawing. By changing the length of one of the pendulums, the patterns drawn will reflect harmonic ratios.

A similar device is made by placing a small mirror at the tip of a tuning fork and aiming a light beam at it. The vibration of the fork can be projected on to a screen and produces a small vertical line. If the the light beam is projected sideways with another mirror, a sine wave is generated. If another tuning fork is placed at a right angle to the first, the harmonic ratios generate ordered spiraling patterns.

Atoms and molecules are subject to constant change or replacement, and yet their angular structure remains constant. Our DNA changes over time and is distinct from other people and organisms, yet the signature helical shape never changes. The chlorophyll molecule that carries out photosynthesis in plants can only do so when configured in a specific twelve-fold geometric shape (that actually resembles a plant). The shapes of the plants and algae that photosynthesize may vary, but the structure of the molecule generating the process is invariate. And *angles* are the functional relationship between two variables that mediate interacting complex patterns.

If you think back to the example of how the flight paths of baseballs hit on a baseball field are fixed functions of time and distance, you can get a sense of the order that is the universe.

This is the reason that **the brain CANNOT be the primary determinant of movement.** The bottom line is that you cannot make things behave any way you want them to. Any and all movements you can ever make will reflect the universal structure and not your whims and fancies.

This is also the reason that **having a brain is NOT intrinsic to the function of movement**. Literally.

The universe tends toward structure. Clumps of dust and ice and assorted particulates come together to form planets and galaxies. Sunlight absorbed by earth (and all its creatures) becomes structured material. The absorption and conversion of sunlight (as opposed to the reflection) is why the surface of the earth is not as hot as the sun that heats the earth. And all of the structures that emerge move according to universal laws of motion. The wind and weather patterns, ocean tides and waves, the motion of the earth itself are all reflective of angular modulation.

Compared to the power of tsunamis, tornadoes and hurricanes, human movement is very small. But this size differential hides a tremendous secret! And that is that **all** movement is derived from *angular modulation* . The distinctions in appearance are due to differences in *scale.*

The scale may vary, but the function is identical.

The constituent components may vary, but the function remains unchanged.

Once there became contrast in the universe, there came angular modulation - a difference in angular relationship that we experience as both structure AND motion.

Let's presume that first there came polarity (energy contrasted into positive and negative form).

From this original contrast arose orderly structured relationships. The force of attraction or repulsion between two contrasting charges is directly proportional to the product of the two charges and is inversely proportional to the square of the distance between them.

This interaction generates a current and electric current produces a magnetic field.

Electric and magnetic fields vibrate harmoniously at right angles to each other generating electromagnetic waves.

Particles of energy, standing waves, organize themselves according to polarity; and when these "atoms" combine to form elements, again it is in a specific geometry determined by energetic angular relationships. The chemical properties of molecules and their interactions is determined by these energetic directives. What you have then, is an unbelievable number of possible forms, structures and flowing changes that all arise from the simple interaction of contrasting forms of energy.

There can be no discussion of any complex or emergent phenomena or behavior that is not based on very simple angular relationships.

This is **symmetry.** Under whatever principle you operate, this principle must hold true for *everything* throughout the universe. In other words, **there is no special or unique way of moving that is strictly the domain of human beings.**

However we move must apply to birds, fish, bacteria, proteins and atoms and so on.

Not everything in the universe has legs or similar appendages. What you need to see is that arms and legs are *expressions of angular modulation* and are not simply flesh and blood limbs.

Moreover, movement is not just angular changes alone. **Movement is a product of the coefficient interaction of angular modulation, friction and earth's acceleration**.

If you lack any in any of these things, coherent, productive movement is impossible. Friction and earth's acceleration are fairly self- evident; you don't get too much done if you're slipping and sliding on a slick surface or if you are free floating in the zero gravity atmosphere of space.

People very much underestimate the importance of angulation. Consider : if you stand upright with arms hanging by your sides, you're fairly "straight" – exhibiting minimal angulation. Now try to move **without making any angles**. Don't press into the ground with your feet. No leaning or bending your knees. No twisting. You will find that **any movement is impossible** !

You can think, wish, pray – send any brain command that you want and you still cannot budge a single millimeter.

Flex all of your muscles to your heart's desire! No movement will be produced!

I've told you some of the reasons why the brain cannot be the commander of movement. We also need to lose the idea that *muscles* are responsible for movement. The whole concept that your brain tells your muscles what to do is stupid from the outset!

If your brain requires an intermediary, then it does not have direct control; it can only offer suggestions.

If your muscles need someone to tell them what to do every step of the way, then they, by definition, have no control. And any organizational structure that controls through intermediaries is an emergent *social convention* and not a universal function.

It may sound as if I hate the brain, but I do not. What I despise is the misrepresentation of the brain. The true strength, the power of the brain lies in its **loose connections**. It is this loose structure of very weak links that allows us to freely associate patterns – to create new connections. **THIS** is imagination and adaptability and creativity. **THIS** is the power of thought. The very thing that gives us our ability to think in ways unmatched by any other creature is the reason that the brain cannot be in direct charge.

Your brain takes information from different sources and then it mixes, matches, and associates and sometimes connects this information to other pieces of information. Some information is filed and stored. Some information is used as a comparison so patterns can be detected.

There really are no rules as to how information is handled. That is the beauty of the system; nothing is pre-organized.

The brain is mainly concerned with *extrinsic* information. Extrinsic information is the meaning that *you* supply to an experience. *Intrinsic* information is information supplied by examination of the thing itself.

For example, if you examine an object, and you experience that it is flat, solid, has rounded edges and is red in color, this is intrinsic information. That it is a stop sign and you have to come to a halt when you come upon it or that it signals danger or restriction of some kind is extrinsic meaning.

Movement that you label a " bench press" or " running" or" brushing your teeth" is actually an extrinsic definition. The angular modulation, the friction and effects of earth's acceleration that form these actions is intrinsic in nature.

You can see that the domain of the brain is extrinsic in nature in how the body is represented in the brain. The parts of the body that are predominantly mapped are the ones that deal with interpretation. The photons striking the retina is brings information that must be interpreted – what are you seeing? Is it dangerous? Can you eat it? So the eyes have a lot of brain area devoted to them.

The same goes for the hands. The information provided by the hands delivers a tremendous amount of information about the environment. So, too, with the feet.

The limbs and the trunk, on the other hand, function in ways that require strong, direct activity with no room for variation. If the trunk and limbs were based on loose associations (like the brain) we would be too "rubber-limbed" to act effectively with our environment. The fine motor skills of our fingers is based on the strong foundation of the limbs and trunk.

So, if the limbs and trunk have to be so stable in function, then why do we have to rethink the role of muscles? Because people are terribly mistaken in their ideas of how muscles truly work.

First off, let's literally get rid of muscles. Imagine the skeleton with just enough connective tissue to hold it together, like those skeletons displayed in (some) doctor's offices and hanging in biology classes.

You can grab hold of the skeleton at pretty much any point and move or swing it around and the limbs would exhibit angular modulation. You could hurl it to the ground and the interaction with the surface would create angular changes. The point being that you don't require muscle to achieve angular relationship changes.

If this sounds stupid, let's use an example with the muscles intact.

Most people assume that the biceps raise the forearm to form a 90 degree angle (more or less), like a "bicep curl ". But identical angulation of the arms is seen in the performance of the Olympic style lift- the clean and jerk. The difference of note is that in the clean & jerk, the angulation of the arms arises from the action of the lower body angulation. Bicep participation is incidental if not accidental.

As with the brain, I don't mean to diminish the function of the muscles, I simply want to bring their perceived role more in line with reality.

It's a mistake to try to attach fixed, absolute definitions to the world of appearances. For instance, someone will discover that adjusting foot position when doing the leg press will make their leg sore in new places. The easy assumption to make is that those muscles must be responsible for movement. Not so.

The angulation is the moving function. The muscles supply power to achieve angulation and conserve angular relationships. **This does not imply that the muscles are the prime movers!**

Let's use the motorcycle as an illustration. The functions of movement on the motorcycle are a built-in feature of its structure; it leans, it rolls, the handlebars rotate freely. If you were going downhill, you would have all you need to ride. The engine provides power to these functions – the engine magnifies the effects that already exist. The muscles in your body act in a similar fashion.

Now is a good time to sum up what I've been trying to illustrate so far and where I'm going with all this talk of atoms and molecules and cosmology.

The physics that describe the universe from its beginning must also be able to describe human movement.

To say that your brain controls movement or that your muscles do any lifting is as naïve as insisting that the sun is a fiery ball that is pulled across the sky every morning by a chariot being driven by some god or another.

At this point, we start getting into movement itself. We discussed the beginning of movement with contrast and angulation. And we should understand by now that there is a corresponding solid structure that is inseparable from the fluid form of that structure.

Now it's time to understand that the universe is not some lifeless form of mysterious energy.

The universe is alive.

We don't have to figure out how or where life "began" in the universe when we grasp that the universe was never "lifeless" to start with. Anything that exists now, has ever existed or will ever exist is simply an expression of a potential that has always been.

So when molecules form amino acids and amino acids organize into proteins and proteins organize into cells and so on, all this self- actualizing is an expression of the "life potential" Inherent in the universe.

This is somewhat of an application of Occam's Razor, which basically states that entities should not be multiplied unnecessarily. In other words, the explanations requiring the fewest assumptions are most likely to be correct.

Instead of a bunch of very complicated theories about the "unique and mysterious" neuromusculoskeletal systems, we're better served by looking at movement from a universal perspective.

We know how atoms and molecules use electromagnetism to arrange themselves (move about). But for motion with greater effect, a higher expression of organization is required. So here molecules organize themselves into amino acids and amino acids fold and link into structures we call proteins.

"Protein" derives from the word "protean", which indicates something possessing a varied nature or the ability to express different forms.

Protein is not just a food group. Protein is more of a descriptive label for a primary function.

Proteins indicate a very broad category of molecules that perform an endless variety of activities. There are *tens of thousands of different proteins.* And it is here that organic movement begins.

Proteins work to process energy – generally by grabbing, releasing and manipulating molecules to arrange and release (wave) energy. In this way, they act as neurotransmitters, cell receptors and even certain hormones. Most enzymes are proteins.

Proteins also transmit electricity (like turbines) and also act as transmitters of mechanical energy (tension and compression). If you were compared to a house, proteins would be the building materials, the construction workers and the tools used by the workers. Proteins would even provide the plumbing, electrical and communication systems.

 Proteins are so swamped with work, so they need help to be effective. Since proteins are elemental – basically super molecules, they don't self-replicate. So proteins make cells which are able to do two things in particular : Make proteins and make copies of themselves. It would be like you building a people making machine that would not only make more people, but would also make more people making machines.

More specific to movement, proteins combine to form appendages used for movement both inside and outside of the cells.

Inside the cell, they are used to re-arrange stuff within the cellular matrix. Outside the cell, proteins form wiggling arms or hair-like "tails" that propel cells around (like sperm cells). Often referred to as cilia or flagella, or pilli, these appendages form the hairs that line your nasal passages and ears and help move foreign material out. They also work in your ears to transmit sound and detect changes in the angular position of your head.

The polymers that are at the root of muscular activity are actin, myosin, dynein and tubulin. This is going to be grossly simplified, but you'll see that more technical understanding is unnecessary.

All non-bacterial cells contain actin and myosin. These are not particular only to muscle cells (Muscle fibers are really elongated cells). Actin is a protein that is active in maintenance of cell shape and muscular activation. Myosin is an enzymatic protein that can split ATP molecules to release energy.

Tubulin is a protein that polymerizes (links) to form long structures called tubulin. Dynein is an enzymatic protein that works on tubulin in a "ratcheting" type of action to generate motion in ciliary and flagellar action. Dynein is an ATPase, which means that it hydrolizes ATP into ADP (and phosphate).

Let's look at how this fits together.

The tubulin and dynein form miniature "muscle fibers" on a sub-cellular level. Actin and myosin are the large-scale cellular version of the dynein/tubulin structure. Basically, The "ratcheting action" I mentioned goes like this: two elongated structures (actin and myosin) align with each other , but not evenly. Between them are cilia-like "arms" that sort of link together and "pull" on each other to align the structures. This aligning is what is referred to as "muscular contraction".

But this image is misleading. When the ratcheting action occurs, molecules of ATP are split to release energy. This energy release and the aligning of fibers work together to form motion, which is enough to do work on a micro level (cellular). But on a macro level (the human being), you need a force amplifier.

This force amplifier – the entire medium for the force generated – is the connective matrix.

Before going into the connective matrix, I want to talk a little more about ATP, which is often mentioned when discussing muscular activity.

ATP is, generally speaking, THE primary form of organic energy. But there is more to it. There is a connection to the cosmos that needs to be understood and appreciated.

To start with, all organic life is made of some combination of Carbon, Hydrogen, Oxygen and Nitrogen (CHON for short). These elements are the first to be formed in the universe. Not only does CHON form all organic structures, **it also forms the energy that is used!**

Creatine phosphate is simply CHON (Phosphorus is related to nitrogen). While ATP (adenosinetriphosphate) is CHON in a more complex structure. ATP is not just energy, it is also part of your overall being as DNA.

DNA is basically comprised of four molecules called nucleotides that join to form a chain called nucleic acid. The four nucleotides are referred to by the letters, A, C, T, and G.

The A is a combination of Nitrogen and Hydrogen that form a molecular base called adenine. If you then add a phosphate (phosphorus and oxygen) and a sugar (carbon), you have a nucleotide.

If, instead of carbon, you add more phosphate, you get a form of energy. Two additional phosphate groups yields ATP, while adding one extra phosphate makes ADP (adenosine**di**phosphate).

The thing to take away from all this is that :

1. everything is formed from the "stuff" of the cosmos
2. "life" arises from the arrangement of this cosmological "stuff"
3. The same stuff that makes living structures also makes the energy used by those structures

There is really no difference in the fluid and the solid forms. Everything is conversion.

The thing about the human body is that context is everything. Remember, we represent a *nonlinear* system. This is why it's senseless to speak of "pulling" or "pushing/pressing" movements as if they were conditions that exist independently of a global context.

The identical angular position of your arm can affect either a "push" or a "pull" depending on the angular relationships and behavior of the rest of your body, particularly the angle of the torso and the and the angular velocity of the legs and pelvis.

Angles. Angles. Angles. Yes, it's all angles. Remember, angulation is representative of the original contrasting function that created everything in the universe. That is what separates this book from every other "exercise and training" book out there. I'm demonstrating the universal symmetry of the principles and ideas that I'm setting forth. I'm not just presenting you with some new activities with which to fill your allotted "exercise time". If it only works in the gym, it's no good. It has to apply everywhere, all of the time and under any conditions.

Back to the importance of context. Imagine that you are riding a bicycle. As you go from a seated position to standing while you pedal, your arms go from pulling to pushing depending on the angular activities of your torso and the pressure of your pedaling action. Then, as you pedal, the bike starts to lean from side to side. And with each angular change, your arms push, pull and at times do both at once (as stabilization) to the point where it is impossible to make a distinction among the actions.

This all due to the collections of loose associations and distributed networks that is our system of movement. Behavior expressed in one phase tends to be little help in understanding transitional behavior.

If each segment moved independently with many degrees of freedom, then any action would have an infinite number of possible effects. And describing the simplest of motions would involve infinite variables.

Each segment, however, is not independent; every action is dependent on local conditions (like adjacent activity). Complex movements are coupled together and rythms overlap, compete and interfere, generating higher levels of energy. Meanwhile, underneath all of these changing conditions, there is a quality that is conserved – angles.

Before any serious consideration can be given to the muscular system, there are some fallacies that have to be straightened out.

- First of all, there is no such thing as the musculoskeletal system. The **muscles DO NOT connect directly to bone anywhere in the body**.
- Muscle groups **are not directly connected to each other**, either.
- Individual bundles of muscle fibers are not directly associated.

Muscles **are** associated through the connective matrix, called the myofascia when referencing the muscle and connective tissue system.

There is a wonderful reason for the muscles not connecting to the bone; If they did, they would comprise a *linear* system , where small changes would only yield an equally small result with no global influence or resonating effect. This sort of system would be severely limited.

For you to be able to enjoy the entire, diverse spectrum of physical activities available, *a nonlinear* system is required. This is the only way that small changes can produce disproportionately large, even surprising, results.

Nonlinearity is what allows a person of smaller dimensions to remain competitive with people who are physically larger.

One other thing must be understood about muscles. The muscular function *must be symmetrical*.

In other words, muscles cannot work one way in one part of your body and a totally different way somewhere else. Your hair behaves like hair no matter where it is on your body. Skin is skin; even if the role it plays changes, its essential nature does not. Whether sensing something or providing friction, its properties don't change .

The same symmetry applies to your muscle tissue. To understand the essential behavioral properties of muscle, let's look at the heart and the muscles of the digestive system. The muscles perform the same function – *they pulse*.

If we examine the actions of actin and myosin, it would resemble the action of interlacing your fingers and unlacing them repeatedly (you can easily see that this short, pulsing activity is in no way large enough to act as some sort of "pulley and lever" system around which most exercise systems are based).

So, if muscles act through small pulses in the heart and digestive system, then they are going to exhibit the same behavior in your biceps. This is symmetry.

Then how do these small pulses generate large, emergent effects like lifting heavy weights or running or climbing?

The answer is in the connective matrix.

Before looking at the human connective network, we have to examine the role of aggregation in organic life. Basically, aggregation refers to a collection of units forming a single body, but can also indicate a number of parts having a loose association. Both definitions can apply to the human organism.

In organic aggregation, the associative material (sometimes called a biofilm) is a living and active participant in the functions of the individual units. It would be comparable to a living chessboard that interacts with the pieces and has an effect on the overall unfolding of the game.

A wonderful illustration of this is microbial aggregation, which is the way that individual microbes can organize and act as an undivided whole in order to accomplish things that would not be possible as discrete units (do you see the relation to muscle fibers and the myofascial system?).

Microbes will cling to a surface and then start to create a biofilm by secreting a viscous substance that forms a shell around themselves. Other microbes will come around and stick to the shell and join in the goo-making process. The microbes then arrange themselves according to individual properties as well as group needs. Even different species of microbes will live together side-by-side cooperatively. The biofilm also allows the different species to communicate with each other! This would be like a biofilm allowing a hamster to communicate with a shrub!

Microbial biofilms are micro-habitats. They even have channels running throughout the structure that act to supply nutrients and form communication links that allow signaling molecules to circulate freely.

The "aggregating substance" that comprises the human organism is much more complex and greater in scope than any other biofilm.

Like the microbial biofilm, the human aggregate is a highly interactive entity. But unlike the microbial habitat, our connective system takes on different forms and changes consistency (while maintaining its organizational power). The best term for this is *connective matrix*.

Specific interactive subsystems will sometimes have their own names, such as myofascia being used to describe the connection between the matrix material and muscle tissue. But joining muscle to muscle and muscle to bone is not the only function of the matrix.

The connective matrix changes consistency and form so that it can be globally pervasive. To that end, it is comprised of many different elements. There are water-binding proteins as well as insoluble protein fibers. There is ground substance like chondroitin and keratin and elastin and much, much more.

Blood is a form of the connective matrix. Along with blood elements like red and white cells, osteocytes, lipids and so on, the liquid plasma serves as a connective function that delivers nourishment and information sources (like messenger molecules) and is also called interstitial fluid. You may notice the similarity to the microbial biofilm.

The connective matrix also forms membranes. These membranes surround, connect *and form* every organ (without it, the liver would spill throughout the abdominal cavity). The matrix also takes the form of the fluid surrounding organs like the heart.

On a smaller scale, the matrix forms cell membranes as well as the environment both inside and around the cells.

During embryonic development, the nervous system is formed from connective tissue and the specific wiring (structure and function) of the nervous system is done by matrix molecules that direct neurons to particular destinations and arranges them once there.

The matrix cells constantly interact with and are inseparable from the nervous system. Matrix cells act as mediators for specific molecular interactions and work to match particular transmitters to their target cells. Matrix material coats every nerve and is designated as the *perineural* system (the neural and perineural systems are flip sides of the same coin).

The perineural system is reflective of the connective matrix's role in movement and is closely associated with motoric processes. Disfunction in the perineural system can take the form of polio, Parkinson's disease, multiple sclerosis and neuropathy.

A great number of neural cells are directed to the cranium and once there, connective material arranges the population of neurons in a precisely detailed structure. And as in the liver, connective material provides a stable scaffolding without which, the brain would spill about like runny custard.

Without a structure, not only would the brain not hold together, the neural activity would become confused. An example of too much neural association is a phenomenon called synesthesia. Effects of synesthesia appear as a mixing of sensory experience. A person might perceive colors when seeing numbers. So seeing the number five might trigger the experience of red. Four would bring on yellow and so on. Or a synesthetic might see numbers when hearing specific notes or tones. For some people, hearing music will actually stimulate the seeing of shapes that correspond to different notes.

At this point, I must reiterate something: **the descriptive labels and explanations that we use to communicate ideas and concepts are NOT to be confused with the actual thing or experience**.

Specifically here, just because I use the term *connective matrix* does NOT mean that the function or expression of the matrix substance is strictly *connective*. It would be just as accurate to refer to it as the *formative* matrix — especially when you consider that the matrix determines specific cell function.

The matrix forms an adhesive substance that glues or binds cells into the particular shapes necessary to carry out their functions. For example, epithelial cells that line the mammary glands will only produce milk when they are formed into a certain hexagonal shape.

The reason I use the term *connective* in conjunction with the matrix is to denote its role in global unity; it is the expression of that which makes us a unified whole. This brings us to the next step in understanding how we work — **a uniform language**.

I had mentioned previously how a biofilm allows different species of microbes and bacteria to communicate with each other. Our human connective substrate expresses a similar function; and the structure of our uniform language is **electromagnetism**.

Electromagnetism (EM for short) , more than anything, displays the symmetry of the universe.

Geometry is a solid form of angular modulation and the first thing to express angular qualities was contrasting polarity (EM). I mention geometry here because space is solid; it has a specific structure that can be measured in distance and/or time (they are inseparably reflective of each other as I illustrated with the baseball field/ fly ball example). EM is the stuff that geometry is made of – at least as far as we can tell, since EM is a manifestation of something unknowable.

EM structures atoms and bonds molecules and in the form of *electrostatic force*, creates clumps of material in space that eventually form planets.

Plants use the EM from sunlight to split atoms of Hydrogen and Oxygen, releasing the energy from the atomic bonds and converting it to a chemical form (ATP) for immediate usage or then further converting the ATP into carbohydrate form for storage.

Humans consume the carbohydrate form of converted EM and transform it back into chemical form (ATP and creatine phosphate) for fuel *and* a biological form – our DNA.

That is correct! We are made of the very same *energy* that the entire universe is made of! Moreover, note that it while our physiology is comprised of other substances (like amino acids, and various vitamins and trace minerals), the guiding force of our human expression is EM/ universal stuff in the form of DNA.

This is why the expression of DNA is not fixed and takes unbelievably diverse forms – it is literally a manifestation of an infinite universal potential. All living creatures share similar DNA because we are all representative of the same single entity.

We have to speak a little more of plant life before going on. Plants convert EM into chemicals for various purposes. Plants can make themselves smell appealing or unappealing. They can use chemicals to attract insects useful for pollination or when being attacked, can release a chemical that attracts the attacker's predators. When in distress, a plant will chemically signal other plants in the vicinity to release chemicals used to protect themselves.

Plants can choose to be edible or poisonous. It would not be inaccurate to say that plants make themselves more appealing to humans so that we will cultivate their presence. Before you scoff at the notion of plants manipulating human behavior, consider the mood changing effects of intoxicating or narcotic plants or the mind-altering effects of psychocillibins ('shrooms). Much of what we know about pharmacology we learned by studying plants.

In the same way that you could see chickens as an egg's way of producing more eggs, you could say that people are plants' way of propogation and expansion.

The most important thing to take from this is that chemical messaging (like hormones and pheromones) are forms of EM.

What we've seen from looking at the function of plants (from a universal perspective) is that everything is some form of the universe and that form is based on EM. But to become a living cosmos, the once unknowable singularity formed distinctive contrasts. The bottom line is that energy requires structure and structure is a form of energy. They are distinctions without any real difference; there is no matterless form or formless matter.

Because everything is an expression of the one thing, there is a symmetry that relates everything in the universe. This symmetry shows up as *non-scaling recursive functions*. In other words, the same processes show up everywhere repeatedly, and in different forms regardless of size. Since scale doesn't matter, there has to be some unifying function; and for our universe, that function is timespace expressed through geometry. Simply put, everything arises through *shape*.

When a plant communicates by releasing a pheromone, that chemical is a molecule with a distinctive shape that is experienced as smell. When a cell in our body expresses as a liver function, it is because the cell takes on a particular shape and along with other similarly shaped cells, are organized into a specific "liver form" (shape).

A messenger molecule in our bodies will have a distinct shape that will be read the same way by different systems. For example, a peptide that means "conserve water" will cause fluid retention in the lungs, liver, kidneys, skin, nasal lining, etc. – a shape being universally recognized.

In the human form, movement generates information in the shape of waves. While wave shapes express geometric dimensions, they are fluid and have a strong tendency to rearrange through interference. This property makes them highly responsive due to their extreme sensitivity to change. Something this fluid must be balanced by an equally high degree of organization.

This necessary organizational structure cannot be a fixed shape since it deals with motion. The elegant solution that is the human movement system is *fixed angulation*.

Fixed angulation is pretty much what it sounds like - our movements are expressed through a series of small angular changes. No part of your body moves beyond a range of about 90^0 before another angular change occurs. *This change does not have to be directly adjacent to the prior angular change*. For example, once my forearm goes through an arc of 90^0, the next angular change can occur at the upper arm, pelvis or feet and lower legs.

Another illustration of the fixed nature of your movements is that you use the same angles to perform everything you do; brushing your teeth, blocking a punch, preparing to throw a pass, eating a cookie, driving a car – all involve basically the same arm motion. You think of these things as different only because you think in terms of their categorization and not the actual expression of movement.

Our movement being a nonlinear system, we are highly sensitive to changes in initial conditions. This can be observed in our hand function; our hands and fingers are extremely limited in their range of motion. Because of this the smallest changes in hand/finger position can generate huge changes in the actions of the rest of the body. Experiencing wrist locks and small joint manipulation (in martial arts practice) will demonstrate this beyond any doubt.

That brings us to the next point, which is that *shape converts energy into a form of communication*.

On a global level, our movement derives from angulation, and the energy that is generated/mediated through angulation requires a medium and that medium is the tension/compression in our connective matrix, and the energy is in the form of EM. This may sound a bit confusing, but I'm attempting to explore the elements of a nonlinear system while maintaining a sense of undifferentiated wholeness. Because when all is said and done, angles, tension, EM, the matrix - are all inseparable aspects of a single event.

Here, we can see the nature of language at work; while it makes it easy to communicate with others, it is also all too easy to mistake the symbol for the thing and thereby create a false separation – a false "reality".

I mention the false separation because as we examine the human movement system, with all of its contributing elements, we are forced to treat these components as separate entities even though they are simply multiple reflections of a singularity – many facets of a single jewel.

So, as you read further about EM and the connective matrix, keep in mind that these subjects (as with all of the subjects in this book) are not separate, overlapping subjects but are **distinctions of an undifferentiated whole**.

On the surface, the connective matrix appears to operate as a system of continuous tension. Imagine a skin-tight covering over your entire body with fibers that attach to every cell in your body so that the slightest local movement anywhere affects your being on a global basis. Add to this "bodysuit" analogy that repeated movements will "thicken and wrinkle" the suit in such a way that your future movements will be limited to fit the patterns that have been created.

Now, there is some merit to this image, but it is vitally important to realize that the tensile nature of your connective system is the underlying structure of the EM language that informs every system in your being, in much the same way that plants release pheromones that transmit knowledge.

Stressing any part of the connective substance deforms energetic atomic bonds. The "excited" electrons generate waves of EM energy/information. The EM pulses inform cells and functions throughout the body (think back to how interfering waves of light on holographic film carry enough information to create multiple three-dimensional images from any section of the film).

The hologram is an extremely simple example of how EM waves **are fluid information** and can be converted to a solid structure. But from this simple example we can see how plant activity (photosynthesis and phosphorolation) can be seen as a form of holography by converting pure EM information (sunlight) into chemical forms (ATP and saccharides). The thing that people too often overlook is that EM carries with it the intelligence of the entire universe.

Since people consider DNA to be the "carrier" of the information required to become "you", and DNA is constructed from a universal incarnation (CHON in the guise of ATP), it is no great stretch to think that plants (through photosynthesis) carry the information for life on earth. And even though humans require protein, the animals that are our usual source of protein are themselves plant consumers.

Plant activity is but one example of the transformation of EM into various forms of information.

Keep in mind that EM in its most basic form is just a contrast in charges which then formed into waves. But in order to have a more definitive effect, a more solid structure is required. Think of it like this : someone giving off "bad vibes" has an effect on you. Someone bouncing a rock off your dome has a more definitive effect!

This EM transformation does not occur through some unseen "magic"; there is an understandable structure. To begin with, electric current is the passage of a charge through a conductor, which carries a difference in potential (positive on one side and negative on the other). Conductors can have the properties of a solid, liquid or gas.

Electric charges also possess a self-organizing, magnetic property – with opposite charges attracting and like charges repelling. This provides you with an instant axiom that can guide bonding and motion. This simple relationship dynamic between charges is a recursive function and will be seen at all levels of the universe and in various systems in the human form.

Each cell synchronizes with other cells and changes its own behavior according to EM changes. Not only do the molecules that comprise the cells possess electromagnetic charges, but the cells themselves act as conductors of electricity. A neural cell's inner membrane has a negative charge because there are more positively charged ions on the outside of the membrane. During neural activation, ions from the outside channel inside, so the inner surface changes from negative to positively charged. Since charges must always balance, the energy from the ionic change generates a wave of changes throughout the entire system, all at the speed of light.

As the cellular membrane acts as a conductor, the connective matrix itself forms a system that generates an electric charge when compressed, twisted, or distorted in some way. Structures that display this property are called *piezoelectric*. Piezo comes from the greek word meaning "pressure" and piezoelectricity is EM generated by pressure or tension.

Generally, when pressure is applied to a surface, a negative charge develops on one side of the surface while the opposite side acquires a positive charge (like the cell membrane). As pressure is applied, an electric charge flows across the material. The electric current changes direction of flow depending on changes in pressure application.

Collagen molecules will orient according to the flow of charges (along lines of tension – wrinkles in your "bodysuit"). Changes in polarity will also cause positively charged calcium molecules to be attracted to the negatively charged surface of bone.

Cells called osteoblasts lay down new bone material according to concentrations of electric charges. Cells called osteoclasts clean up old bone material while avoiding the new material by detecting differences in electric charges. Even the earth's acceleration (gravity) and atmospheric pressure act to stimulate piezoelectric charges in bone material. This is why astronauts who spend time in a weightless environment suffer loss if strength and bone density (as do people who don't get the proper sort of exercise).

When considering bone material, it is important to realize that bone is part of a continuous connective system and its distinction is that it expresses a more solid property than the other forms of connective substance. But bone is not that hard, calcified thing you see when you look at a skeleton on display. What you see there is bone material with the collagenous substance baked out of it. If you were to take bone and dissolve the calcium salts out (using an acid, like vinegar), you would end up with a bone having the feel and consistency of a piece of leather.

Bone is not just enmeshed in connective tissue such as cartilage, ligaments and tendons; all of these things are but expressions of a single connective function (we just have to treat them as distinctions to understand their roles).

Bone is surrounded by different densities of connective tissue with greater density at the ends. Connective tissue (in the form of endomysal fibers) associate each muscle fiber with its surroundings. This allows the coordination of each fiber's activation with the activity of its associated connective material. So each centimeter (for example) of angular change in the bone will be accompanied by a muscle fiber activating.

A couple of different things can occur with each pulse of muscle tissue. As with everything, there is both a physical movement and a corresponding energetic form. When a muscle cell pulses, it ratchets together. When it does so a phosphate group is split from a molecule of ATP and a bit of energy is released. The pulse of energy is a pulse of information, a ripple traveling at the speed of light.

But the ratcheting pulse of movement also acts as a miniature tectonic plate shift. At the bottom of the ocean, energy released from a tectonic shift would generate earthquakes, undersea landslides and tsunamis. Within our "sea of connective substance", a wave (tsunami) of myofascial tissue is generated . For instance, when you flex something (say your bicep), the "muscle" moves in a little wave.

Every point on a wave front can act as a new source of waves. And wave interference can be either constructive or destructive. As I had talked about, anything can be transformed into a wave pattern and EM waves can carry a surprising amount of information (as with the case of holography).

EM waves as information is how the brain both communicates and receives information. The brain has no direct contact with the world - it possesses no "blueprints of correctness". Information is already organized when it reaches the brain. Now, once the brain has a good amount of information stored away, it can make associations and connections and re-form the information it has. The brain can then send out its own waves and interact with the rest of the system, creating a *resonating organization*.

The brain is only a single element in a complex system. It can recognize information, store it, categorize, recall, or rearrange it– but it is not the *originating* source of information.

I went through the discussion of plant functions to show that EM waves aren't just *carriers* of information – **they are a form of information!**

In the plant, splitting H_2O into Hydrogen and Oxygen releases energy that is then reshaped into stored energy or information (pheromones, for example). In the human being, molecules of ATP are partially split (forming ADP) and energy is released. This energy is shaped by angular modulation and intensity of generated EM, thus becoming information that will be processed by the brain.

To illustrate the ability of angles to become information, I'm going to make a stretch and compare the human function to writing on paper.

The letters of the alphabet are formed from small angular shapes. These shapes in a particular order form words. The words occupying a specific positional relationship on the paper form sentences and paragraphs. And at some point (which differs from person to person), these word structures generate ideas – the words stop being simple carriers of information and actually *become information*.

Our connective matrix plays the role of paper – a timespace structure for organizing and solidly shaping information in the form of angular modulation (including EM).

Section Two

The vast majority of people display a child-like, almost primitive understanding of timespace and motion as some simple "cause and effect" happening. The average American's conscious grasp of physics goes something like this: "Mongo hit ball. Ball go up." Or: "Mongo push bar. Bar go up."

As a matter of (sad) fact, this pretty much sums up every "sport science" and "high performance athletic training" program on the market – "mongo push hard on ground, Mongo jump high. Mongo do again (and again)". Spectacularly stupid.

Even so-called "biomechanical" explanations simply replace a mystery with a label and pass themselves off as "knowledge".

For instance, how does your arm really work? The "biomechanical" explanation is to tell you that your arm is a *class two lever*. But what the hell is a lever? A lever is a label that covers a broad category of functions that alter the angular relationship of time and space. The function is the important thing – not the image of a crow bar that probably popped into your head.

So, the answer to the arm question boils down to the expression of the energy converted when there is a change in relationships that include time/space, tension/compression and electromagnetism.

It all sounds so complicated, but the good news is that because this is a universal function that applies to everyone, everywhere and all of the time, you don't have to "know" this; you don't have to understand physics to fall down –

physics is operative no matter how ignorant you may be. But if you want to know how to use the ways of the universe to improve your life, then you may want to expand your understanding of how the universe works.

No one said life was easy.

The purpose of this book in general (and this section in particular), is to strip away the misleading images and notions surrounding movement that are actually detrimental to your performance.

To do this, you must come to understand that the concepts and labels that you use to think about movement are *abstractions* – they are cognitive techniques used for the filing and transferring of information.

Also, remember that the label on a file is not the information contained in the file and the information contained in the file is not the actual thing that the information describes. What you have is different levels of abstraction.

Now, you can apply new and different labels to files and you can store additional information in the files, but that won't make any meaningful changes in the actual thing to which the files and labels pertain.

Your brain, as far as movement is concerned, is a *filing system*. It labels and stores and transfers information, **but it does not perform the actions that generate all that information**!

Your brain indirectly receives pre-structured information and what you experience is an abstraction of the actual event. For example, what you experience as "smell" is based on the interaction of specifically shaped molecules with the molecules in the linings of your nasal passages.

To become so entranced by abstraction is a particularly human trait. This is why we value an impressionist painting of a hillside more than a tourist's photograph of the same locale. It is also why humans spend so much effort in looking for shapes in clouds, clothing stains and wood grain patterns.

This instinctive need to find and apply patterns demonstrates that the brain does not *control* this activity, but rather that the activity is a *triggered response* – like when seeing one thing suddenly reminds you that you forgot to do something else; or when seeing something triggers an inappropriate response, such as an innocent gesture triggering anger simply because you associate that gesture with someone else that you don't like.

Your brain is just as easily fooled by motion cues, such as experiencing the sensation of motion when you are stationary simply because you see the vehicle next to you move. *Perceptions are fluid* and change according to context and additional input. Perceptions and your brain's tools of perception (vestibular sensors and such) are used to accurately file incoming information, but are not intrinsic to the actual movement.

Bats and scorpions don't perceive the world as humans do and yet they still move just fine. Bacteria have no human cognitive skills or awareness and they, too, still move – **and**

the basis for their movement is exactly the same as it is for humans. Gravitational timespace in the form of tension/compression rules *everything*.

To demonstrate that you already know this, we'll use a motorcycle as an example. I used this example earlier in the book, but you probably skimmed over it. However, it is important and bears repeating.

If you are traveling at a modest 15 MPH and you turn your handlebars to the right (at about a 45⁰ angle), you will travel in a short arcing path to your right. Now if you are traveling at 50 MPH and you turn the handlebars the same as you did before, the arc of your turn will be much different. If the angle of the handlebars is constant, the arc of your path is inseparable from your speed, no matter how hard you "muscle the turn".

Staying with the motorcycle example, all the movement functions are intrinsic to the structure of the motorcycle itself – if you don't put the kickstand down properly, movement will take place. The engine itself isn't necessary for motion – it only puts the "motor" in motorcycle; the cycle is able to move without it. Your brain is like a fancy computer in a computerized motorcycle engine – it is able to sense fuel and air interaction as well as speed and electrical stuff . But these are added features and are not the things that comprise motion. Even within the engine, the computer can influence combustion within that motorcycle but the computer has nothing to do with the actual chemical reaction.

Labels and concepts are of little help in making meaningful changes in your performance. This is because labels and concepts are NOT what took place and you can't make changes in something that didn't happen!

Much of strength training makes use of the concept of leverage. But, again, this is a concept that delivers no real understanding. A lever is a label that describes the interconnectedness of time, distance and angular modulation (fulcrum position). My point is that if you only have a lever "label" that conjures images of prybars, you have gained no understanding at all because time, space and angular modulation governs **ALL motion in the universe** and not just that of simple machines.

The human brain is a late-coming intermediary. Cognition is not intrinsic to directed movement. Some creatures respond to or move toward chemical stimuli (this is called chemotaxis). There is also phototaxis (response to light) and magnetotaxis (response to magnetic fields) as well as elasticotaxis, which is response to physical tension.

Creatures that are not as cognitively oriented as humans are able to swim, walk and track prey right from birth. The more cognitively skilled the creature (the more the brain acts as a middleman) the longer it takes to integrate movement skills and the brains activity. Dogs take a little while to learn to catch a Frisbee; it takes humans much longer – some humans never master the skill.

The fact that in many instances our brains stand between stimulus and response makes us slower, but we do get to think about why we are slower.

Really, the act of catching a Frisbee is more the domain of phototaxis and elasticotaxis. The actions of your eye muscles and neck as you track the Frisbee as well as the changes in light qualities expressed by the moving Frisbee is the information that guides movement prior to or even without cognitive input. You don't require a " tiny person" inside your head rapidly performing complicated mathematical calculations.

As a matter of fact, we've all experienced conflicting thoughts wherein we argue with ourselves or criticize our performance. So if there are little individuals in our heads, they obviously cannot agree on anything and therefore could not possibly be considered to be "in control" of even the simplest of matters.

It is going to very difficult for most people to simply get rid of their dependence on what they think and believe. So I'm going to address some specific errors in thinking that seem to be the most prevalent.

Athletic trainers (and sport science) in general struggle to formulate motion into a linear equation that can be easily explained - sort of a "calculus of human movement".

Calculus basically describes a rate of change in some variable using differentiation and integration. Before you start protesting that you don't do any differentiating an integrating, I'm obliged to point out that this correlative math is at the heart of every exercise program in America. When you lift weights, the weight used corresponds to the amount of resistance you can overcome while moving in a specific range of motion ; it is NOT, however, an indicator of "strength" or the ability to move in multiple ranges of motion simultaneously (like in real life). The same goes for counting reps and measuring your waistline – these are *symbolic* of a correspondence and should not be mistaken for the actual function of human motion.

So, back to calculus. Differentiation is finding how quickly something changes – the rate of change of a rate of change, as opposed to the average overall rate of change. Integrative calculus finds the future values of a variable by summing (integrating) the rate of change at each instant.

The problem with this approach is that it assumes that any curve (rate of change) is going to be smooth. Since Isaac Newton's time, mathematicians have furthered that assumption by believing that any curve with sharp angles (sharp changes in behavior) could be split into separate, smooth sections that could then fit the methods of calculus. Today's fitness experts fall victim to the same assumptions in the way they approach human movement.

Unfortunately for them (and for those that they train), this approach is doomed to fail because the method of separation (divide and conquer) only works when phase shifts (changes) are definite, identifiable and predictable. The human motoric system is dynamical, nonlinear and resonant – precisely the kinds of details people want to leave out when trying to present a clean, neatly-packaged system or viewpoint.

Human motoric function is not *governed* by time, space and gravity (timespacegravity – TSG); it is *reflective of* TSG. However.... Within the human system, there are highly unstable coefficients that make us nonlinear *and* unstable – chaotic, even. In addition to the usual suspects like friction and momentum, these elements also include mental state, emotional arousal, perceived effort level as well as fatigue and pain threshold – even the type of footwear you choose will have an effect on your performance. So, even within a fixed and stable structure, we can express patterns that are *aperiodic* – regular and if not *un*predictable, never repeat exactly.

Your movement is without a steady state unto itself. This is because it's an association of events that can have multiple critical points that magnify seemingly small changes. And the nonlinear quality means that such critical points can show up anywhere in the system.

Human motion is complex and emergent; it's also undifferentiated, overlapping and interdependent. But for all of that, there is some quality that will be conserved throughout any possible changes that the system may undergo. That property is *angular function*.

Imagine (or go out and try for yourself) standing and holding a weight that is too heavy to simply lift or "curl" with your arms alone. The weight is such that no amount of muscular strain or positive thinking will move it. So what do people naturally do in such a situation? *They make angles!* They bend their knees and lean forward and then arch back as their legs straighten. We've all done this and have seen it done in gyms everywhere. The strain and the direction of

the effort of your mind and your muscles changes
throughout the lifting process, but the function of angular
modulation is reiterated.

You might think with all the angular orientation that motion can be described or formulated geometrically. It cannot. The human in motion is not describable in terms of Euclidian geometry because of the nonlinearity factor. In other words, the angles we use are few in number and are uniform and symmetrical; the effects of these angles however, are aperiodic and synergistic (the emergent results will not be equal to the efforts put into the system – for better or worse - and you can never say exactly why).

The main reason (geometrically speaking) for this is that our angular modulation is *fractal* in nature.

The word *fractal* comes from the Latin word *fractus* which means fragmented, discontinuous or broken – exhibiting an irregular form.

The important thing to know about fractals is self-similarity; It expresses some quality or feature that is reflected at every level of a structure no matter the size or position. A head of cauliflower is a perfect example. If you break the head in half, you can observe that each half is comprised of smaller versions of the whole head. If you snap off a smaller piece, you can see that the smallest pieces also are just tiny versions of the whole.

The human body is also composed of many interlocking, self-similar shapes. For example, a muscle group displays a "cauliflower-like" fractal structure; The muscle group is comprised of bundles of myofibrils (fibers), which contain bundles of sarcomeres, which contain bundles of myosin/actin polymers – all nested within each other at smaller and smaller scales.

The magic of fractal geometry is that it allows bounded curves of infinite length as well as closed surfaces that contain an infinite area. For example, draw a triangle. Now, attach a new triangle at the middle-third of each side of the original triangle so that you have three new triangles identical in shape but a third of the size. What you have now is a "star of David" shape. Keep adding triangles to the sides and you end up with a snowflake shape (called a Koch curve). You could keep repeating this procedure and what happens is that each transformation adds length to the design while the total area remains finite.

A similar effect can be made by expanding area. Take a square and divide it into nine equal squares. Now remove the center square. Keep repeating the procedure on all of the remaining squares. This is called a Serpinsky square.

In biology, this sort of fractal expansion is called *bifurcation*. This process is important because it allows the packing of a tremendous amount of functional material into a finite area. For example, the human circulatory system squeezes a huge surface area into a finite volume. This is not just a space-saving feature; Remember that blood is part of the connective matrix and delivers nourishment and information. So in most tissue, no cell is ever more than three or four cells away from a blood vessel. The lungs consist of millions of bronchial branches that are packed within the connective membrane which allows them to function as a whole.

You also see bifurcation in the branching of trees. This allows the trees to expand into a large area without a corresponding increase in weight. Our bones do the same thing for the same reason - we get area without needless extra weight.

Both the human form and function are made of many, many interconnected self-similar systems. It can all be very confusing because if you were trying to separate the human being into discrete sections, you would not be able to clearly categorize the transition from one phase to another. Anatomists try to understand the human being in pieces and parts and go about labeling stuff, like classifying blood vessels according to size – arteries, arterioles, veins, venules and so on. But even anatomy texts admit that the transition from one category to another is not clearly defined; Some intermediate arteries have walls that suggest larger arteries while some larger arteries have the structure of smaller veins.

Categorizing misleads; The fixation on apparent features obscures the symmetry that exists across the imposed sectioning. For instance, hurricanes can be understood as a continuum of smaller vortexes that do no more than swirl trash around in the street. In biology, the structure and function of motion can be found intact across species – from microtubules to flagella to fins, legs and arms – self-similarity abounds.

Self-similar patterns also apply to energetic expression, such as heart activity. The fibers of the heart muscle that carry pulses of electricity have a fractal form and so do the pulses that they carry. Exertion levels, heart rate changes during exertion, each heart beat and the biochemical changes that reflect each beat all form self-similar waves superimposed on each other.

It's important to understand how expansion "into space" also displays a fractal geometry. In nature, you see this expansion by adding identical, but smaller, sections in the growth of seashells and the horns of goats and sheep. This expansion method is also called aggregation. The aggregation will also either narrow into a line or form a spiral shape as they narrow to avoid instability and breakage. The interesting thing to note is that they will follow a universal pattern called the Golden Ratio, or Phi. This pattern of growth is also seen in flower seed patterns, leaf growth and the helical form of DNA.

Crystals build up by self-similar aggregation. Crystallization consists of tiny duplicates of what will be the final form connecting to form the whole structure. In snowflakes, for example, water freezes, then the crystals form extensions that grow to a point of instability where they then branch out in another direction. Now, when water freezes, the molecules form hexagonal (six-sided) shapes. Like all crystals, the whole is the same as the constituent parts, so *every* snowflake is hexagonal – having either six sides or six points.

The point of all this is to show you that there is an underlying symmetry – a unifying, universal order to everything ; Nothing is random or isolated.

This pervasive, universal structure means that certain functions, if not easily described, are always available – they are aperiodic, yet invariant in general. It is free will within a deterministic universe. It gives you realistic choices in its limited structure. It's much easier to choose from a three-item menu than it would be if you were given a menu with a billion choices. You would starve before you could even read through the appetizers.

While movement itself doesn't require a "brain", a brain is part of our function as human beings. Cognition isn't necessary but it is inseparable for us. The thing to remember is that our brains don't create information out of nowhere, it already exists in some structure and the brain simply "reads" what's there. And as I have painstakingly explained, nothing simply " pops into existence" independent of anything else. And all this interdependence will have a symmetry that is not constrained to any single category.

To keep things extremely simple, if not entirely exact, we'll consider the universe as contrast that takes on two distinct forms – time/space and electromagnetism. In the human body these two forms appear as connective matrix (time/space) and chemo-electric energy (electromagnetism). Changes in the connective matrix is reflected In chemo-electric changes and vice versa. The format for these changes is tension/compression. Tension and compression are two terms for the same event – they are flip sides of the same coin. For instance, if you stretch a rope tightly by pulling on the ends, you apply tension but the fibers of the rope are being squeezed together – compression.

Tension displays the property of self-organization, or as Hooke's Law of Elasticity states: within the limits of elasticity, the extension of an elastic material is proportional to the applied stretching force.

And all that tensing/compressing generates electromagnetic charges that also self-organize. For example, when a piece of metal becomes magnetized, its charged particles polarize. And if you cut a magnet in two, the poles don't separate – each half reorganizes to form two complete magnets.

Simply rubbing a piece of metal with a woolen cloth can magnetize it (a connection between tension/compression and electromagnetism). And if a conducting wire goes through a surface at a right angle, a magnetic field is generated where lines of force are concentric with the wire (an illustration of *directional* self-organization).

So you can see that information is already structured before the brain receives it; and technically it was never *un-*structured, since matter/energy/structure can never be created nor destroyed – it can only change forms. The information was never unstructured any more than time/space was unstructured before the human brain came along.

The purpose of all this is to get rid of the confusion and myth surrounding things that people were aware of thousands of years ago, but have since been forgotten. The knowledge was passed on through many cultures but had to be in a general format that could transcend language barriers. Unfortunately, people became fixated on the format of the information and forgot all about the intended message – fixating on the pointing finger instead of glimpsing what the finger points to.

Let's look at breathing. Breathing is touted as the connection between the conscious and subconscious – presumably because it's an involuntary function that can also be voluntarily affected. This represents a truly superficial grasp of the underlying functions.

When you hold your breath, there will come a critical threshold – a breakpoint – where you can no longer continue to hold your breath. With practice, you can extend the length of time before this point is reached. But this offers no real insight.

But hold on to your butts! I'm about to drop some knowledge on you.

For far too long, it was believed that the brain, somehow sensing decreased oxygen levels and/or increased CO_2 levels in the blood (via chemoreceptors and sensors) was the controller of breakpoint. WRONG!

First of all, if reduced O_2/ elevated CO_2 levels were the determining factors of breakpoint, then there should be some measurable level that acts as a threshold – a common bottom line. There isn't. And if gas levels triggered breakpoint, then you wouldn't be able to immediately hold your breath again – like with your next gulp of air – because of the time it would take for gas levels to return to normal. Obviously untrue.

Research has also demonstrated that the nerve connections between chemoreceptors (in the carotid arteries) and the brainstem are not involved. With the feedback system disabled, people should have been able to hold their breath until passing out, but this, too, proved untrue.

The answer lay in the tension/compression and electromagnetic relationship between the diaphragm, heart and throat complex (including the glottis, larynx,etc.).

The tensional oscillation of the diaphragm as an influence can be seen when breath holding can be prolonged by moving the diaphragm. And the "blackout" of oxygen deprivation can be instantly brought about by a sharp blow to the nerve complex in the throat (the phrenic nerves, vegus nerves and glossopharyngeal nerves).

The point is that breathing and various methods of breath interruption are illustrations of how information is organized before cognitive intervention and how that information will reflect a universal structure – in this case tension/compression and electromagnetism.

Simply put, the specific angular activity of the diaphragm is reflected in the generated electromagnetic waves that interact with the angles and electrical activity of the throat, lungs and heart. It is the interference pattern of these waves that create the "hologramic" language that is read by the brain.

It's important to understand how this breakpoint works because it reappears throughout the human function – a fractal symmetry.

Most of the time (pretty much the whole time before reading this book), this most essential function of fractal symmetry passed unnoticed by people. This is because the system works on its own and needs no "controller" – no human strain and effort. This is what was meant when people (at one time) were exhorted to "move with the universe" or when it was said that you could only truly express power when your movements were "in line with the universe". These were not some inscrutable words of "Asian wisdom"; these were early physics lessons that were meant to be accessible to every man. At one point in history, physics, chemistry, neuroscience were meant to be helpful and usable to people in general – unlike today, where education is used to separate the "learned few" from the rest of the rabble.

The ancient teachings of Tai Chi, yoga, and zen martial arts practices have always been meant as paths to UN-learning. In the west, the emphasis is on filling the mind with "knowledge" and always **more** – more techniques, more protocols, more programs, more weight, more reps, ever more and more and more. "Wholism" is a dirty word to the western man, who finds security in being able to hang a label on everything (as if naming something were synonymous with actual knowledge). America worships at the feet of the athletic trainer who can name every muscle in the human anatomy (even though any separation is a false separation).

The westerner desperately seeks someone who can train him/her to "move correctly". This is like the fish who is unaware of the water in which it swims. Human movement is fixed, naturally flowing, ever-present, pervasive and supporting. There is no "functional movement" – there is only movement. Searching for a " functional movement program" or" strength training program" is as insane as thinking you are "lost" because you saw your own reflection on the side of a passing bus.

Come to grips with this: There is NOTHING that ANYONE can EVER show you that will violate the movement structure that I've outlined in this book!

The methods used by the eastern man to gain knowledge were based on direct observation and firsthand experience. Western concepts of human movement are built from experiments under controlled circumstances and observations of behavior removed from a natural context.

I'm not being critical just because I'm Asian. I'm merely pointing out what should be readily apparent if not immediately obvious – western athletes display a tremendous degree of muscularity and excel in certain aspects of physical activity; but they also suffer unbelievably high rates of catastrophic injury. I'm not just pointing out that "the emperor has no clothes on"; I'm pointing out that he's had three back surgeries and a pec tear. But is that not the appeal of western sports? It's possible that you will witness an athlete perform a feat of majestic grace and agility. It is equally likely that you will witness the athlete blow out his knee on national t.v.

From a historical viewpoint of history, this sort of "athletic ability" is worse than useless – after all, if you cannot continue a sustained level of performance without crippling yourself, how would you be able to work the land or hunt? How much use would you be on the battlefield? And I'm not just talking about some ancient battlefield in Mesopotamia. If you were a settler or a trapper in the 1800s, your activities of the morning might include killing three men with a knife and a handy sharp rock – and you would still have to go about surviving the rest of the day.

This is why much of the scientific knowledge of the Eastern man was garnered on the battlefield and the science of movement became inextricably linked with martial application.

Let's start with India, the birthplace of martial arts. The people of East India realized that there was a recursive aspect to human movement. And they developed a systemized understanding of this underlying symmetry. We call this understanding *yoga*. But don't picture a bunch of skinny, really flexible guys sitting around while chanting, "Om" (even though "Om" was an early version of "cosmic string theory"). Yoga derived from the practice of warfare. The Eastern Indian was a bad dude – it is from this culture that we get the words "assassin" and "thug".

Yoga was comprised of a limited number of "postures" and the transitions between those positions (there were eight postures if the history books were accurate). These postures made up *every possible* movement a human being would ever be able to make. Eight doesn't sound like much, but think about this: Let's simplify the number of angles your body can express to your arms and legs bending (four angles) and your pelvic motion (twist and tilt- four angles), and your shoulders/upper arm angles (two angles). That's ten angles spread over eight postures. If we could compare this to a combination lock, you would have eight tumbler positions that could consist of any combination of the numbers 1 through 10. Most locks that we use only have three or four positions and that offers a seemingly infinite number of possibilities. So eight is not an unreasonable number.

The fact that you are constrained in your movement angles serves an extremely important function: it makes it possible for small changes to have immediate, global effects. Think about it – the most sensitive parts of your anatomy (hands and feet and genitals) have the least amount of motion available. Other than bending in one direction, your fingers and toe can't move at all, and the bones in your hands and feet move even less. Even the slightest change in these areas affects the entire being.

This can be demonstrated in the effectiveness of joint locks – especially those of the wrist and fingers, which will drop a man to his knees in a millisecond and render him combat ineffective.

You now see that we do not possess the range of motion that you may have first thought. As a matter of fact, it is almost binary in its simplicity – your arm is bent or not bent; your leg is bent or not bent. You have function (bent) or disfunction (straight). Straight is disfunction because you have to bend something in order to move.

The binary structure of your limbs is interconnected. This is illustrated in the "judo" foot sweep. (most people today are unaware of this link, so I'm about to improve the judo technique of countless practitioners).

When you walk, the arm on the same side of the stepping foot move in fixed coordination – as the pressure in your right (stepping) foot goes from back to front, your right arm will (elbow) will pass over the length of your foot simultaneously. If your arms are bent and not swinging as freely at the deltoid, then your hand will travel the length of your foot step.

If I want to "sweep" your stepping foot out from under you, it will be most effective if I sweep at the moment you step forward *but before* your weight settles on to the foot. This is too tricky to try to visually calculate when the right moment will arrive and is the reason so many people suck at foot sweeps. But I'm going to remove the guesswork; since elbow motion is connected to foot step, when I pull your elbow out away from your body, *your next natural footstep will place your foot under your extended elbow*! All I have to do is sweep at the point under your elbow; your foot will be arriving there shortly.

If I were to execute a shoulder throw on you, really all I am doing is extending your elbow and the preventing your natural step by blocking your torso with my body. If I hit you with a fireman's carry (throw), again all I do is extend your arm and prevent your natural step by blocking your knee and "boosting" you across my back.

What you should see here is that what appears to be three totally different martial techniques are really various ways of taking advantage of a single function.

The human form is restricted to limited degrees of motion in any single plane. But remember, it takes surprisingly few constituent parts to generate unbelievable variety – everything in the universe is comprised of only 92 elements in a few simple geometric shapes held in place like magnets.

It "feels" like we move in all sorts of ways and perform an endless variety of actions, but this only seems so to your brain because your brain labels everything as if were a separate thing unto itself. In reality, reaching for a cup of coffee, typing a report, washing your hands in a sink, etc. all involve the same basic angling of your arms. Even reaching down to pick up the morning paper off your lawn involves the same arm motion - the difference is in the angling of your torso (and perhaps your knees) as you angle your arm.

Your brain labels these as different events because that is what your brain does – it gathers information and makes associations. The more information there is available, the more associations can be made. And if information doesn't immediately present itself, your brain will *generate* information – even if that requires creating separations and categories that don't necessarily represent wholistic reality.

You could say that we represent an organization with low entropy; in other words, we can experience very few changes without disturbing our ordered form. This is how we orient ourselves. You may be under the impression that we orient through "stretch receptors" and "load sensors" and all sorts of other proprioceptive sensors and receptors. These sensors *transcribe* information – they do not transform, generate or control the energy that the information describes.

Your nasal passages have receptors that interact with molecules and this interaction generates the sensation of smelling freshly baked cookies. These receptors cannot, however, alter the angular, energetic molecular interaction.

Receptors and sensors are part of your neural system. Your neural system isn't restricted to the brain cells residing within your cranium; you have neural cells everywhere and any cell is capable of making and receiving neurotransmitters. You even have motor neurons in your hand that are active in movements that require immediate action where a global response might take too long. Simply, you possess neural capabilities that do not require tendon receptor involvement.

When you experience pain or discomfort when moving beyond your normal range of motion, this is generally due to the brain's response to the information it is receiving in comparison to the information that it has on hand. The brain can, and does, play a role in our movement – it can enhance or interfere with our efforts. Again, these are *subjective* labels; stretch, load, pain – even "up" or "down" are creations of the brain and are NOT intrinsic to movement. The direction that you refer to as "up" would be considered "down" to someone on the other side of the earth. A satellite orbiting "up" in space might actually be passing beneath your feet.

With that in mind, you can now see that you don't "raise" or "lower" a weight or yourself. You don't push yourself up when performing a pushup or dip – your motion is a reflection of the energy released through angular changes. Now, that is the way that we were meant to function, but because the brain can exert an influence on our performance, people tend to try to maintain the "right" posture or form while performing an exercise and thus impose a needless strain on the system by preventing natural (and necessary) angular changes.

The brain's participation (including pain and discomfort) isn't all bad or unnecessary; it works to keep your brain on the same page with the changes that need to take place. The point where the tendon/stretch receptors kick in will be at the point of angular change; the tendon receptors are just there to mark these changes in the brain's recordings.

Now we're at the point where you can begin to realize that actual information is comprised of energetic transformations that have their own structure – tension, angles, electromagnetism and so on; the verbal descriptions that we carry around are abstractions that *overlay* reality. The verbal instructions that you are bombarded by are essentially useless – and are often *detrimental* to performance.

For example, "running" isn't something you do; the word running describes motions being expressed by you. If you add the term "fast", you've added another level of abstraction by describing a description – another step further removed from reality.

Most of the time, imagery is no better than verbal description (as they are really versions of the same thing). Runners are coached using terms like "thigh drive" and "stride length" or "arm drive"; the problem is that these words are food for *thought* – they are NOT the actual "language" of movement. Thigh or knee drive is a reflection of hip flexor (psoas muscle) activity – but who the hell can feel their psoas muscle? It only makes its presence known through movement. It is comparable to the arch of your foot; the arch has a MAJOR impact on the qualities of your performance, yet you really cannot "feel" the arch except through the pressures exerted on it.

This *expression dependent existence* describes the movement patterns that govern your being – you can only observe the patterns through movement. I'll try to clarify using a geometric example: shapes like squares, circles and triangles are easily identified. But they cannot be identified by observation of their component parts – a piece of a circle doesn't look like a circle; a line doesn't look like a square or a triangle and so on.

Your movements also form shapes and express relationships that are not implied by observation of the constituent actions. This is why static stretching is a waste of time; you're stretching a muscle whose activation will be dependent upon, and relative to, a host of other actions – both local and distal. Its job isn't to stretch (or lengthen); its job is to generate energy as part of a global effect.

Isolation exercises like the leg extension are also (generally) an exercise in futility. In reality, activation of the upper leg structure (extending the leg) will be accompanied by reflective activation *everywhere else in the body*. **Your physiology works as a single, undifferentiated whole**. Forcing isolated activity is dysfunctional, generates uncoordinated movement patterns and is an invitation to poor performance and grievous injury.

If we revisit the circle, it is the entirety of the circular expression that contains the magic of universal nature – all circles exhibit self- similarity; no matter the size, the relationship between the diameter and the circumference will always be the same- pi. So not only does a curve not look like a circle, it will not express the universal nature of self-similarity . When you work muscle groups in isolation, not only do you not express the complete natural pattern that they are a part of, but you also don't activate the global, self-similar angular modulation that *is* human movement.

The other major problem with isolation-type exercises is that angular modulation involves "breakpoints" (like in breath holding). Angular deviation alters tensional levels and at a critical point will generate a phase shift. In other words, one group of angles transforms into another group (or pattern) of angles (as opposed to one angle moving to another in a linear fashion). The angles will be the same, the groupings can be different. This exhibits the *fractal* nature of self-similarity in human movement.

Let's look at what angles I'm talking about. We'll use the arms as an illustration. Your arm (upper and/or lower) has about 90° of rotation – if you extend your arm and then extend your thumb (like you were hitch-hiking), your thumb only goes from thumb up to thumb down in one specific arc (inward in front of you). Your upper arm comes away from your body (to the front or out to the side) to about 90°.

Now, you might be saying, "Wait a minute! I can raise my hand from straight down by my side to straight over my head! That's 180°!" The total range of motion might *appear* to be a 180° arc, but there is a *phase shift* halfway through. In order for your arm to go from the bottom half of the arc to the top half, the angular position of your scapulae (shoulder blades) must change; and this change is reflected in the participation of your latissimus muscles. Hold your arms out in front of you (parallel to the ground) and lock your lats down; you will find that no further upward movement is possible.

Your upper arm can also go from extended out to your side to extended out in front of you – again, an arc of about 90°.

Your lower arm can move up toward your upper arm in about 90⁰ or so of motion (depending on how skinny your arms are).

So, what you have is a certain degree of movement in your arms (the same or similar number of degrees) and a few fixed angles. There is no changing – no amount of flex and strain will move your arms beyond these limits.

As you move within allowable ranges, there will be points where you can continue moving in a certain range, but only by activating other angular changes (as with the scapulae and the overhead reach). You will feel sensations of stretch or strain at these breakpoints. These are "attention" signals that alert you to an impending phase shift that may require greater conscious effort . In other words, *without* a load, the phase shift would happen automatically; but *under* a load muscular effort may be required.

This is the beauty of the fixed relationship! It *frees* the mind! If you had total freedom in range of motion, your *entire* brain would have to be devoted to the simplest of movement . It would take the efforts of TEN brains to keep up with every sarcomere and its activation! The only way that you can make changes in the middle of expressing a movement or do multiple actions at the same time is if the brain is NOT devoted to the execution of each and every action.

Fixed patterns and limiting structures are not a bad thing. It's NECESSARY! If time/space wasn't fixed, a pop fly might go to center field or it could rocket to the moon or it might travel at a rate of two centimeters an hour. The universe expresses symmetry which we experience as predictability- as "solid reality". The symmetry of time/space/gravity guarantees that when you wake up in the morning, you won't suddenly float to the ceiling or weigh 2,000 lbs.

Our existence as humans is reflective of this symmetry. When you purchase a movie on DVD, the entire movie exists in one location in time/space. But for you to enjoy the movie, you have to put it in a player that extends the time aspect. In DVD format, the movie exists in a "single instant" – your perception requires that you experience the movie over 90 minutes or so.

Another way that fixed time/space helps us is in leverage. We know that changing time changes distance and the emergent effects. The obvious example being a simple lever, like a see-saw or a pair of pliers. Less obvious is a knife and a fork, which minimize the time/effort required by minimizing distance/area of application.

We also extend time when we use a catcher's mitt to catch a baseball – the padding and the extended area of the mitt extends the time of contact with the ball so that it doesn't transfer all of its energy to our hand in a single, painful instant. We also add time and distance (area of application) when we recruit two friends to help us push a stalled vehicle – there's contact spread across the rear of the car and each person adds time through their individual effort, even though the effort takes place simultaneously.

Another form of the time/space structure is *gravity*. I don't mean that it is some *separate* form, or even a *distinct* form – I'm addressing it as such because that is the way most people have learned about gravity.

The important thing to understand here is that **you cannot overcome gravity – ever**.

We discussed in the previous pages the importance of a stable universal structure and also how the universe allows for transformations that can mask the stable nature of things with fluid expressions. Case in point – time is a stable and fixed feature of the universe, but it also takes the form of distance and makes appearances as simple machines and various other physical manifestations.

One of the ways that gravity makes an appearance is in curved space, as seen in the earth's orbital pattern. But even if you were in a vehicle that took you out of Earth's curved space, you would still be in space/time – only less curved or curved differently. So you don't "overcome gravity" any more than supporting a weight with your arms is "overcoming " your legs.

You do not overcome or defy gravity – **your motions *express* gravity**.

The Earth's path is an expression of time/space/gravity (TSG for short). The earth doesn't "fall" in toward the sun; the earth moves in a straight line. It is the TSG that curves. When you hit a pitched baseball, there is an energy conversion and the ball's curved path is the expression of that conversion in TSG form.

When you swing a kettlebell, the arc of the swing is part of a conversion of energy generated by angular modulation and that conversion is expressed in curved TSG.

The thing to take notice of in these activities is *that there is NO vertical component in your movements*.

Every move you make is a horizontal angulation.

Think about it: when you raise your arm, it really simply moves forward and back. When you jump "up", you angle your legs by moving your knees forward and your hips back. This stores energy which is released by quickly changing the angular position back; the stored energy is released and is expressed in curved TSG – a jump that actually describes a *horizontal* arc.

The point is that if you are spending your time trying to lift things "up", you are needlessly recruiting muscular effort in an effort to do something that is simply not possible – you are struggling to overcome the very structure of the universe!

You cannot move "upward" because of *your* structure, either. There is no" you" that is above you or beneath you that can pull or push you vertically. In other words, every bone and muscle group is attached in such a way that your spine and pelvis form a center point around which any action revolves. Every action will have a fixed point so **cannot move upward or downward** – you can only make angular rotation.

People used to know this; this is where we get the aphorism that "you cannot pull yourself up by your own bootstraps".

One of the problems that plague people today is a completely egocentric view of the universe. This is how we still entertain foolish ideas like "the sun rises"; the sun

doesn't rise! The earth spins as it revolves around the earth and this is what changes the sun's position as we observe it.

The sun may look to *you* as though it moves vertically, but the reality is that the sun neither "comes up" nor does it "go down".

I'm going to finish this book with some photographs. These are not "monkey see – monkey do" pictures. They are simply meant to help you visualize certain ideas.

The ideas presented in the photos are not all-inclusive, nor do they represent all of the information in this book. What you will see is the starting point for movement – ALL human movement.

The issue that I have with heavily illustrated "exercise" manuals and "how-to" videos is that people simply ape the behavior depicted in the material instead of seeing the reality beneath the obvious appearances.

For example, despite the vast sea of "how to run (or sprint or marathon)" lessons that are available, you don't actually run; you simply express a pattern of oscillating angular relationships – you form angles and return to a base position and the energy released in the changes generates motion. And everyone works the same way (some more efficiently than others). Unless a person has three legs or a spine that moves in a lateral serpentine motion, he will NOT have some "special" way of doing things that is not immediately available to you. You just have to be reminded of the truth and learn to trust yourself; you are a reflection of the universe and as such are total and complete – there is nothing that you need to add or subtract.

I mentioned angular changes. You have a few fixed relationships. And any deviations in the fixed angles will generate information/awareness that affects you as a whole. One of the most basic systems of fixed angles is composed of the arches of your feet, the bends of your inner elbows and at the backs of your knees, and the palms of your hands. The concavity created by the slight bend of the joints (when standing naturally) acts similarly to your diaphragm or your eardrum – disturbances in the tension generates waves of energy. Think of these areas as cell phone transmission towers; the position/location of your phone can be triangulated by cell tower activity. This is how your brain tracks your location and activity – by the waves of piezo electricity generated by changes in tension.

You can picture these waves of energy/information as the ripples generated by dropping stones in a pond. Dropping stones in different places and in different sequences or dropping differently sized stones will produce different wave patterns.

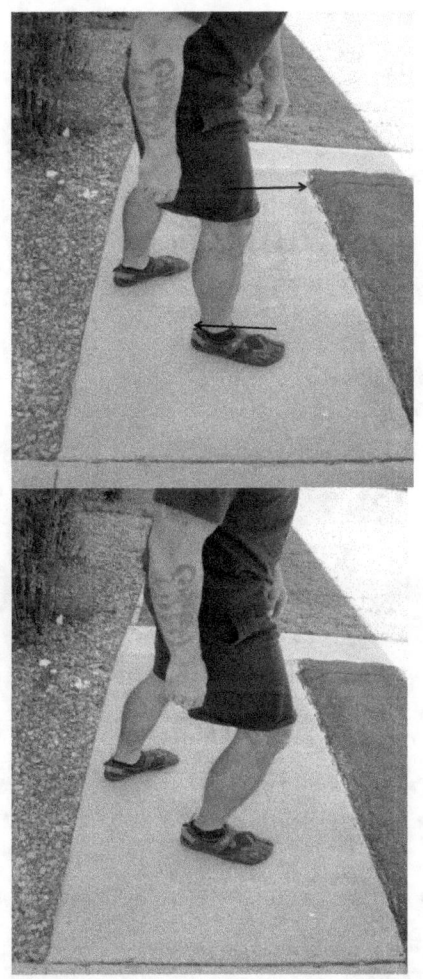

These pictures illustrate the angular function of the lower leg. The degree of angular change will generate tensional changes in the arch of the foot and the connective matrix of the pelvis.

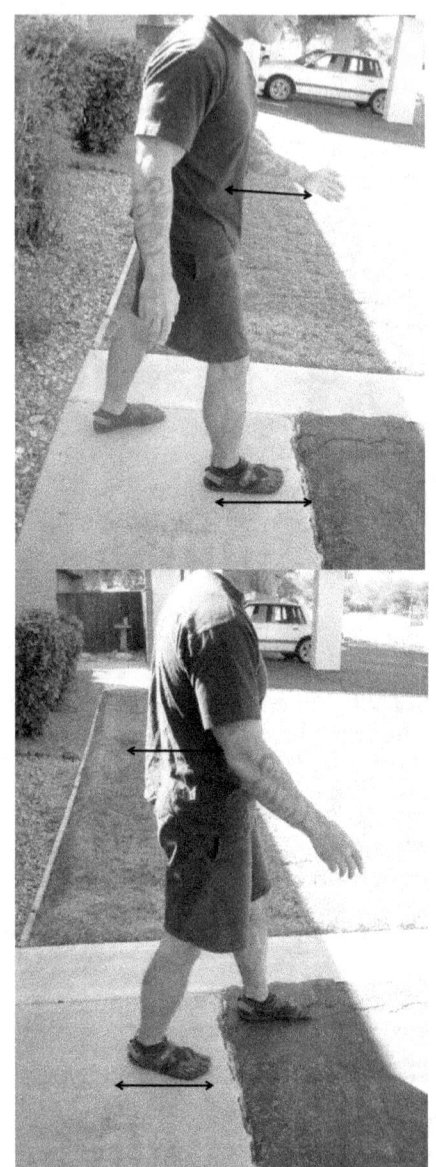

These pictures demonstrate how the arms and legs orient. The hand and the opposite foot have aligning paths as do the foot and elbow on the same side.

This is reflective of the counter-rotation of the pelvis and the solar plexus.

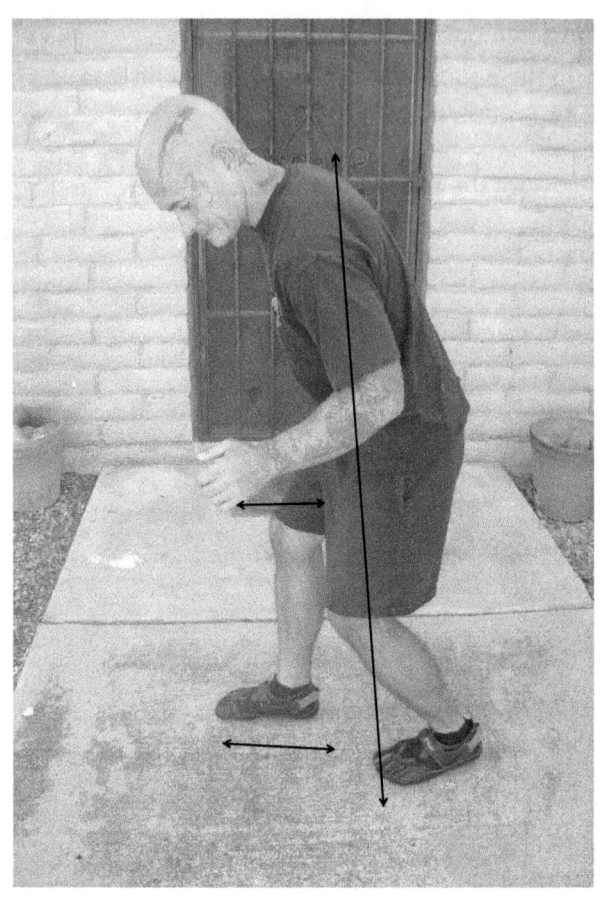

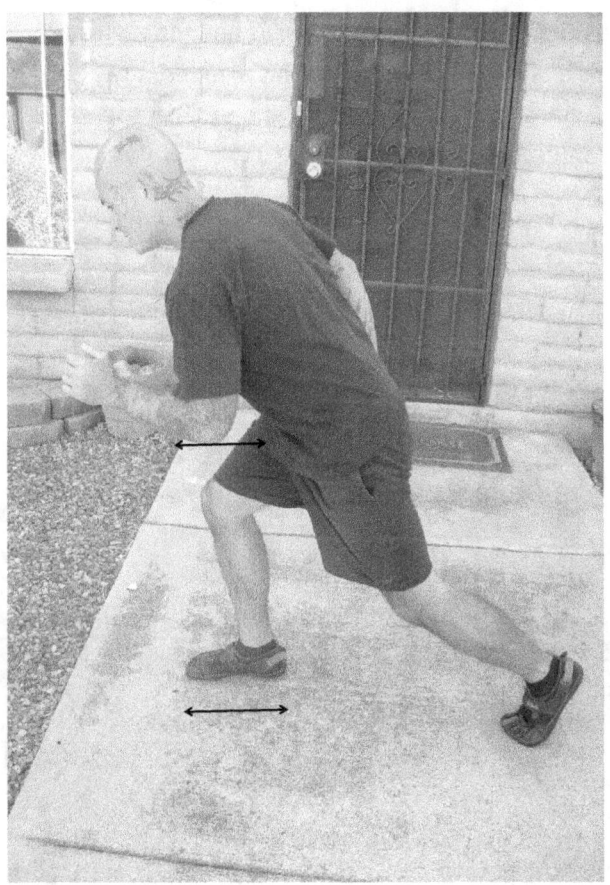

These pictures demonstrate the angular relationship between the hand/elbow and foot but this time note that a more pronounced forward lean alters the angle of the torso so that the opposite elbow and foot will move in alignment (rather than the hand).

Also take note that the shoulder, pelvis and foot will align. The knee's angular deviation from this alignment generates tensional changes which will reflect in piezo electric activity and neuromuscular activation.

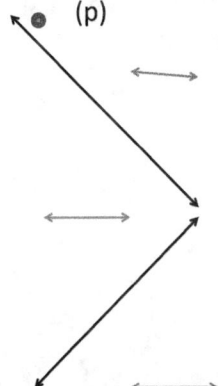

This is an illustration of how you *only function horizontally*. The bones move back and forth and get about 45° of motion at a pivot point (p) which would be at the pelvis and deltoid. Your deltoid moves about half the distance that your elbow travels.

The linear distance that your deltoid travels is the same distance that the pelvis angles back and forth.

When you walk or run, your arm motion helps keep your shoulders and pelvis related angularly. This also keeps your structure aligned over your feet. The angular pressure you experience in the feet also direct the muscular activity involving the pelvic system (hips). The point is that you should be able to see the resonant organizational system at work as well as how movement must reflect the properties of the universe.

The linear aspect of our movement is the space/time/gravity base. The arcing or circular movement we can display is the nonlinear neuromuscular aspect of our movement.

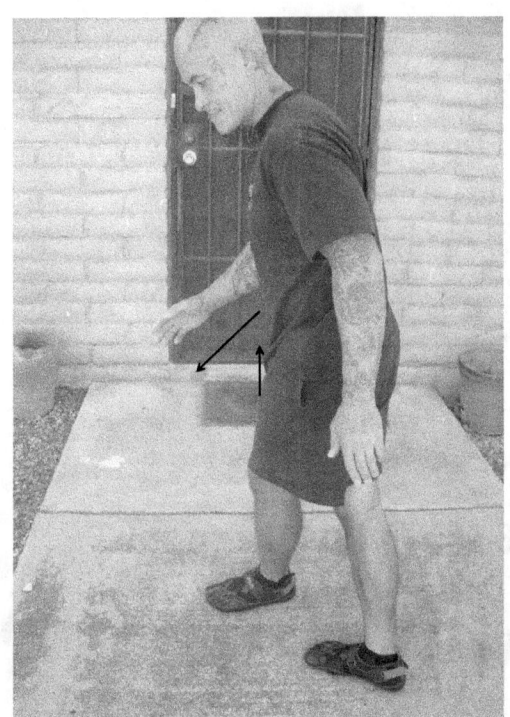

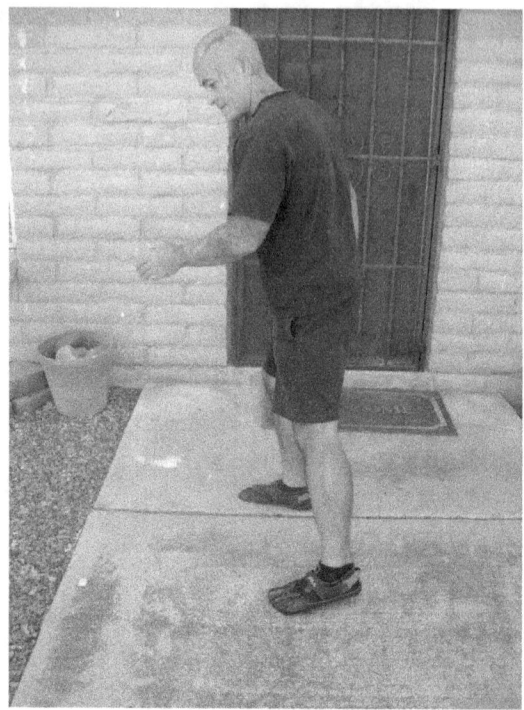

These pictures illustrate how "running is not running". Note that the pelvis moves horizontally left to right. My right hand moves horizontally right to left, across the front of my pelvis. As I make my second step, my pelvis moves right to left while my left arm moves left to right.

My legs do not move "sideways".

They still angle out and back in front of the pelvis – it is the pelvic motion that generates the crossover effect.

Note that the arms move across the front of the pelvis. If you refer back to the previous photos, you will see that the arm movement may align with the feet, but they cross in front of the pelvis also (as the pelvis rotates horizontally from side to side as you walk or run).

This action keeps the line of your center of mass/gravity over the forefoot of the foot that will press into the ground. Basically, your solar plexus, pelvis and pressing foot will align.

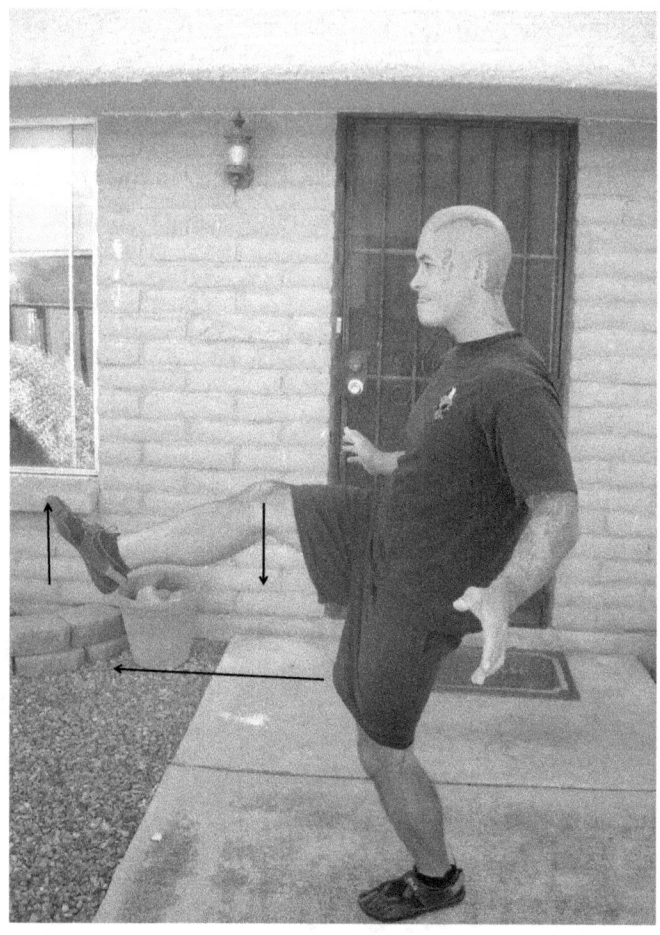

This is a "front kick". Note that the kick is nothing more than a step; as the kicking leg extends, the knee only travels the length of the kicking foot – never more; never less.

If I want to execute the kick with great power, my left arm will have to cross in front of my pelvis as the pelvis moves right to left. Because a kick is no different than a step, the mechanics will be no different.

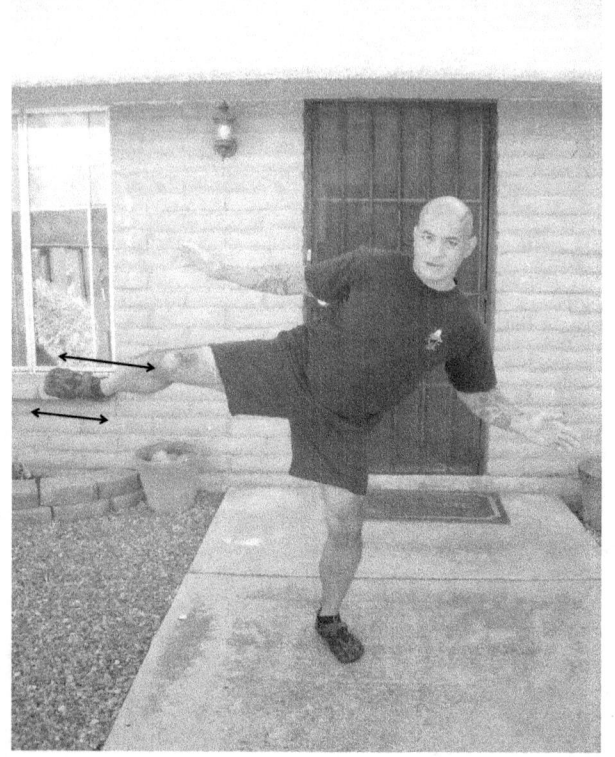

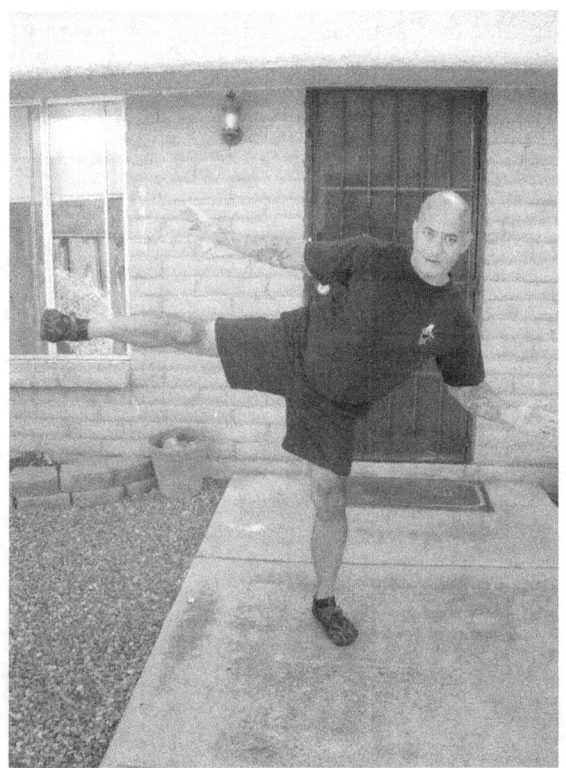

Here, in the "side kick", we see the same knee travel/foot length relationship in the kicking leg (as well as the standing leg).

Of vital importance is to understand that this is as high as I can kick as far as the pelvis/ femur angular relationship is concerned.

To kick higher, I would move my pelvis back as my torso angles forward. This effectively changes my structure to a posture similar to leaning forward in a sprinting "take-off" position.

If I do not lean forward, the pelvic position determines the amount of tension in the "core" area so that I would be limited to the shallower angles used in "walking". If I angle my torso forward, the tension in the core area will be less, allowing more contractile action in the abdominal muscles and greater angular mobility in the legs, like in sprinting.

Though labeled a "side *kick*", the functions are the same as in the front "kick" – and the front kick is no different than walking or running. So in reality, there's no difference between walking, running, and kicking; these are labels of distinction rather than expressing some actual difference.

As important as it is to understand how our various movements are really a reiteration of the same few functions, you must also see how our movements are a singular whole driven by angular relationships; one local angular change is reflected by angular modulation globally.

This exposes the limited benefits of static stretching. When you sit on the ground and maintain a static position to stretch your hamstrings or groin (like in the "hurdler's stretch" or the "splits"), you prevent the associated angulation of the foot arch and the pelvis. The stretch that you feel signals **dysfunction**. Ordinarily, any stretching of the myofascia in the legs is mediated by the angling of the foot and pelvis. In a forced static position, however, the stress is not dissipated and you feel your tissues being stretched. Your muscles, in an effort to correct the overload, will generate energy in an attempt to prevent further insult or damage (remember that your muscles generate energy and do not themselves do any pulling). This is why as soon as you release the stretched position, your myofascia will tighten up even more than they were before you began your misguided efforts.

Stretching in a static position stretches your tissues and snaps them back like a rubber band – great for injuring yourself but no good for "warming up". Warming up comes from the heat generated by the energy released through angular changes – from doing the thing you want to do.

The same " limited benefit" situation applies to most weight lifting-type activities. When you lay on a bench to push a load in a linear path, you prevent any global angulation from taking place. Unless you are preparing for an activity that is limited to the "prone on a bench" position, you are wasting your time. Any pushing-type activity found in life or sports (especially football) is based on **lower body angular coordination**; at NO time during a football game are you lying on your back while pushing a static load in a straight line.

When you cultivate disproportionately large muscles, you are displaying the body tissues' response to repeated dysfunctional movements. Over- loading isolated angular motions creates a situation exactly like static stretching – stress is unable to transform into a global effect. When subjected to repeated isolated stress, the physiology produces more energy- generating molecular structures in an effort to deal with the unbalanced force being experienced. In other words, to keep your joint complexes from being ripped apart, the body produces more muscle proteins – in effect making a stiffer elastic band effect.

The problem is that athletic skill is dependent on the transforming and distribution of stress – not on the ability to deal with loading in forced isolation. Remember, not only is force a form of energy that needs to travel, changes in angular relationships changes in piezo electric activity – broadcasting information that will be used by the brain to form patterns. When you work in discrete "packets" of motion, it is very difficult for the brain to make globally associated movement patterns which are necessary for higher levels of performance in daily activities and athletic endeavors.

This attempt to impose separation and isolation is perfectly illustrated in the obsession with special shoes. At one time, wearing special orthopedic footwear was the mark of some sort of dysfunction or birth defect. Now, these shoes are marketed as "athletic" in nature and everyone has been convinced to wear them – thus becoming a sign of a *mental* defect.

The pressure changes generated by foot angulation is the information that forms angular changes in the rest of the physiology. If these pressure changes are muffled or impeded by footwear, the rest of the body and all of your movements will lack needed information about the environment . This would be similar to poking out your eardrums so that you won't be able to hear the annoying sound that your car has started to make.

Foot, knee and lower-back pain is a sign of dysfunctional movement patterns rather than a need for expensive shoe purchases.

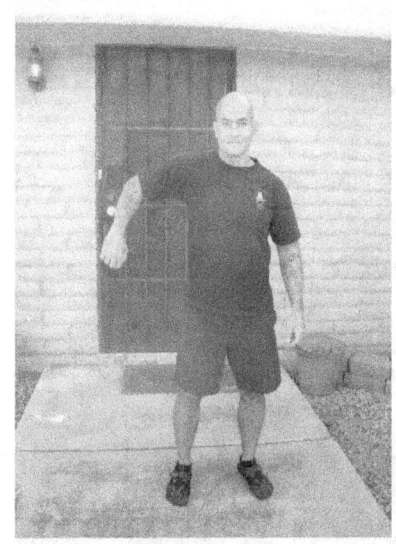

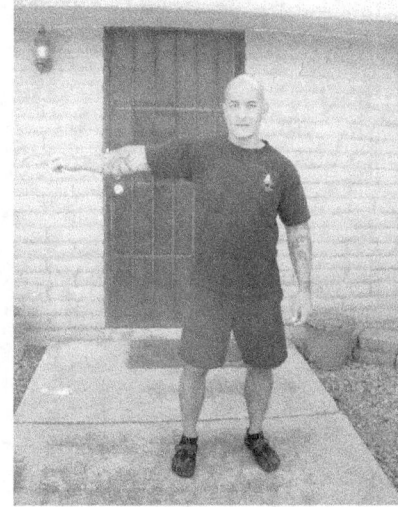

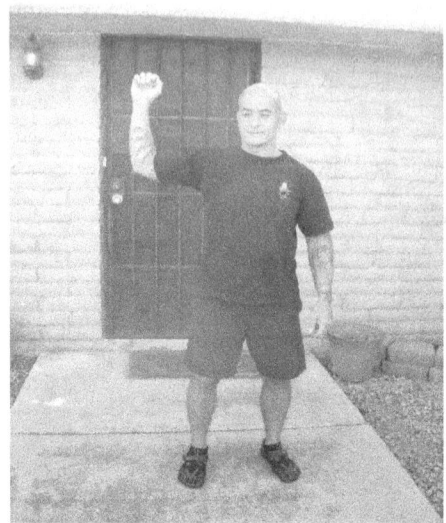

These photos demonstrate what is, basically, the entire range of motion available to your arms. Any other angles will be accomplished by angling elsewhere, such as the pelvis and/or the legs.

If you practice a martial art that includes a knowledge of joint locks, you will recognize these as the positions necessary to secure a straight arm bar and entangled arm locks (figure 4, Kimura, sankyo, kotegaeshi, short-arm scissors, and so on). A large variety if locks and takedowns and "come-alongs" are based on these three arm positions, since these represent the limits of structural mobility.

You will also note that these are the arm positions that are used to throw a baseball or football, write stuff down, pick stuff up and/or scratch your butt.

The variety of movements and activities that you engage in throughout your life will involve some fluid combination of these three positions.

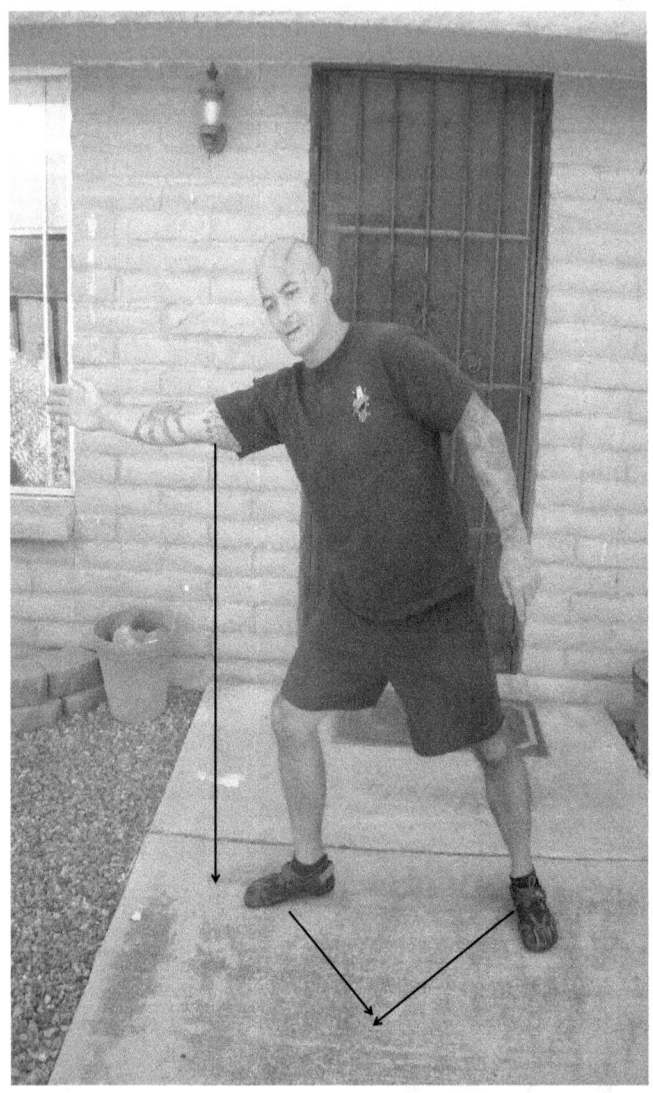

What you see depicted here is the fixed relationship between your elbow and your innate need to structurally align with ground. If I were to be pulled to my right any further, I would be forced to take a step which would land at a point beneath my elbow. If I were to have my elbow directed to the front, the location of my next step would be where the arrows intersect on the ground. If I were to be pulled violently, I may step past that point, but where the lines intersect would be where my butt would land.

This is because your pelvis aligns over your feet, so wherever the foot would land is where the pelvis is going to go. If there is no foot there, the pelvis lands on the ground at that point.

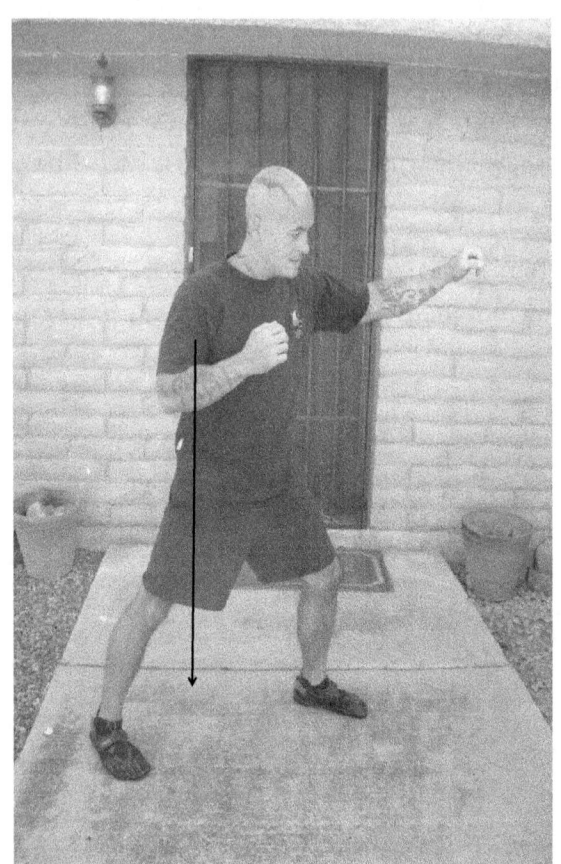

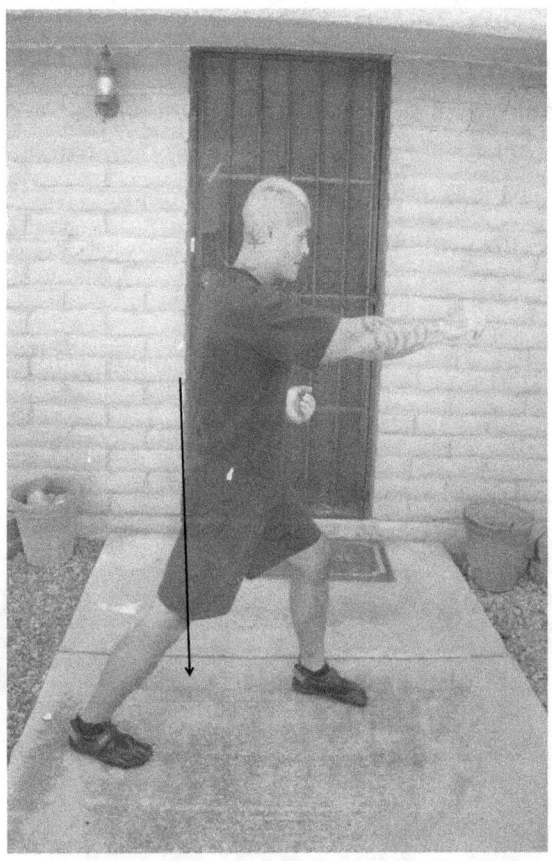

Aside from some really wicked punches being thrown, these photos show the elbow/foot alignment. Also note the tendency of the arms to cross in front of the pelvis, this tendency is amplified to add power to the strike. The only way to extend reach would be to angle the pelvis forward where the sternum would be over the foot (natural structural alignment)or I could step farther forward (because the elbow would automatically try to align over my foot).

Once I notice a person's tendency to punch by either elbow/foot alignment or sternum/foot alignment, then I know how his structure aligns and, thus, I know where his head will be at the end of a punch, so I can slip his intended blow and then bounce one of my own off his dome.

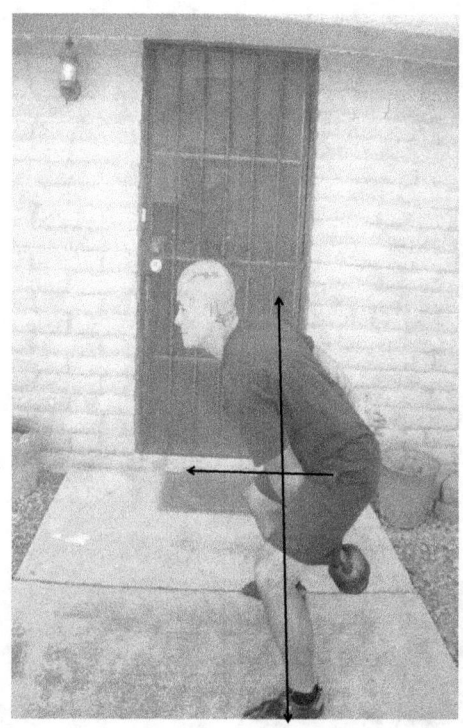

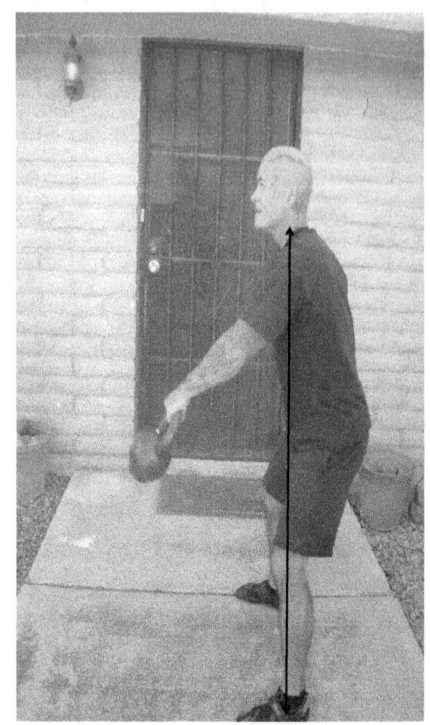

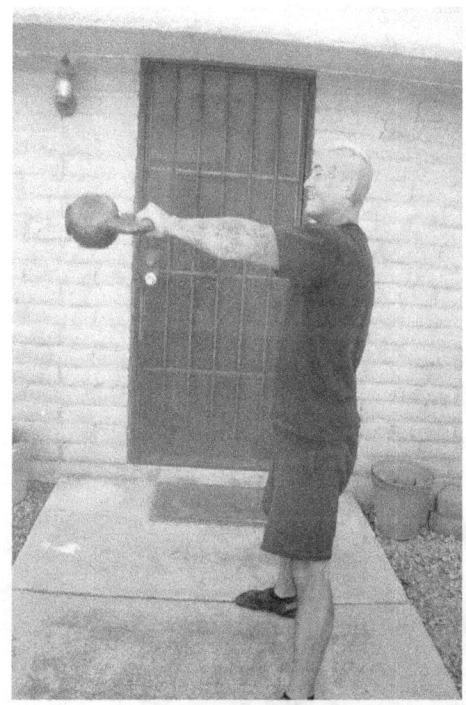

Though this is called a kettlebell "swing", you can now see that it is the exact same alignment that takes place in every photo, despite the perception that I'm performing "different" actions.

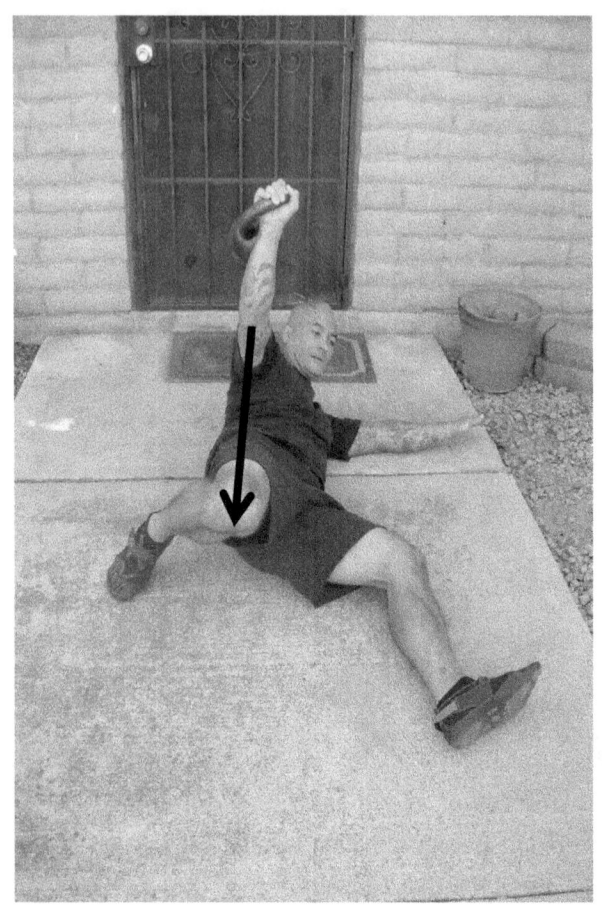

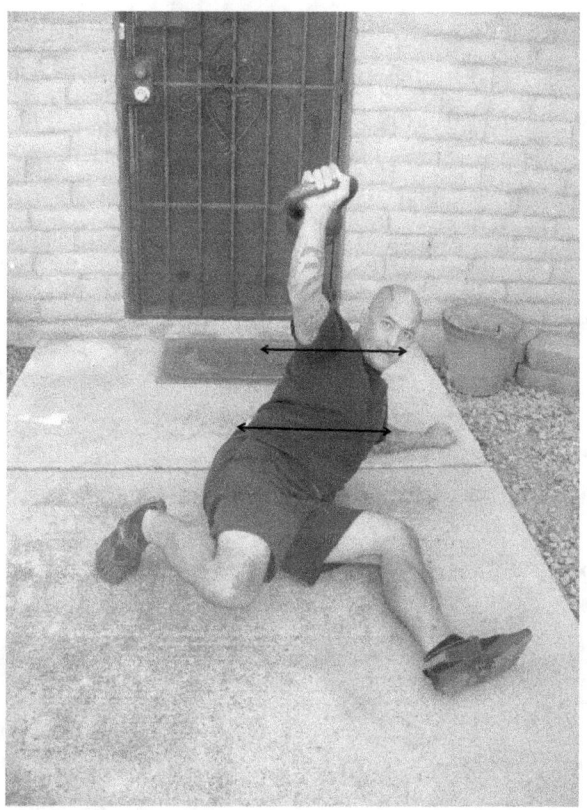

What is being demonstrated here is the tendency to self-organize according to structure *and* gravitational requirements. The kettlebell drops in a line with where my sternum would be if I were to lay back on the ground. As I start to rise (in what is called the "Turkish get up"), my elbows and knees (or feet) will still try to align, even when I am not yet upright. It is actually the process of aligning that directs and generates the muscular force and movement patterns that I will use to get vertical.

Also of importance is to note that counter-rotation of the pelvis and solar plexus work to conserve the gravitational alignment spot.

In other words, if I were to continue getting up without this conservation, my sternum would travel beyond a point of stability, rolling me onto my stomach. The counter-rotation of the pelvis insures that my solar plexus doesn't go too far to my left and all muscular activation will be directed toward getting up rather than trying to stop me from rolling over.

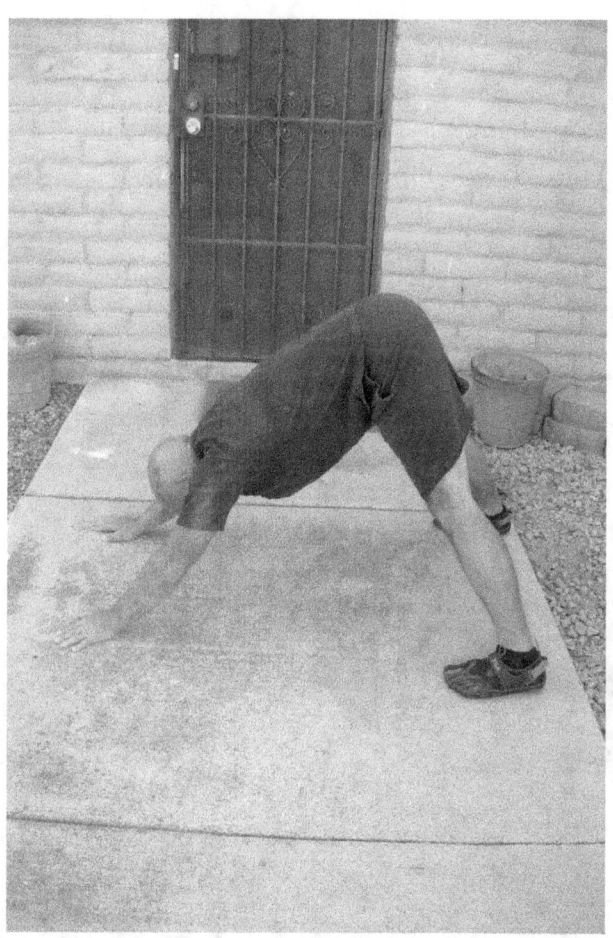

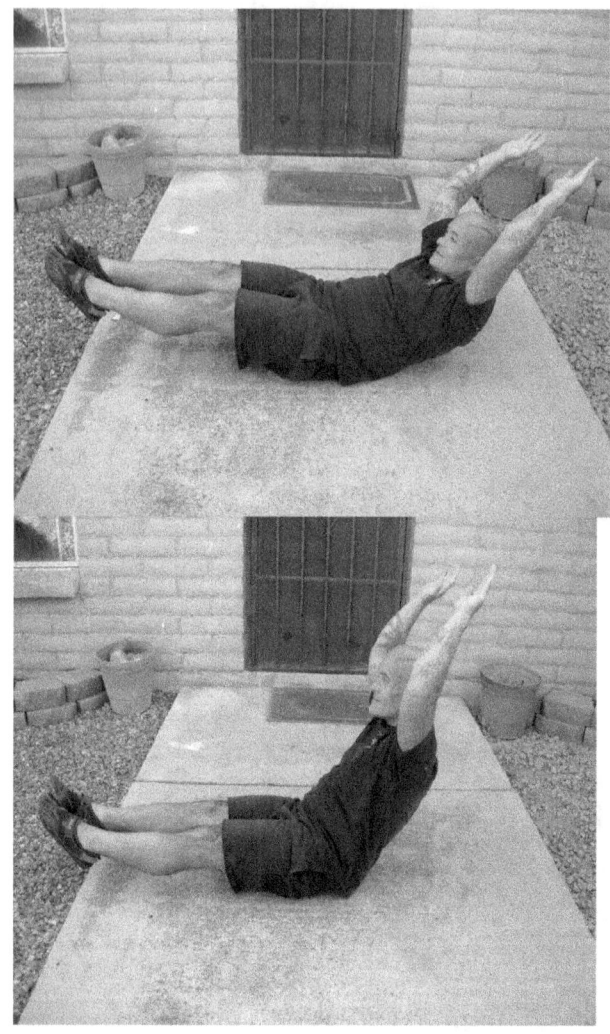

What you have here is an illustration of how the same alignment exists but simply in a different *context*.

Elbows/ shoulders over knees/feet – it's a seated kettlebell swing as far as your connective structure is concerned.

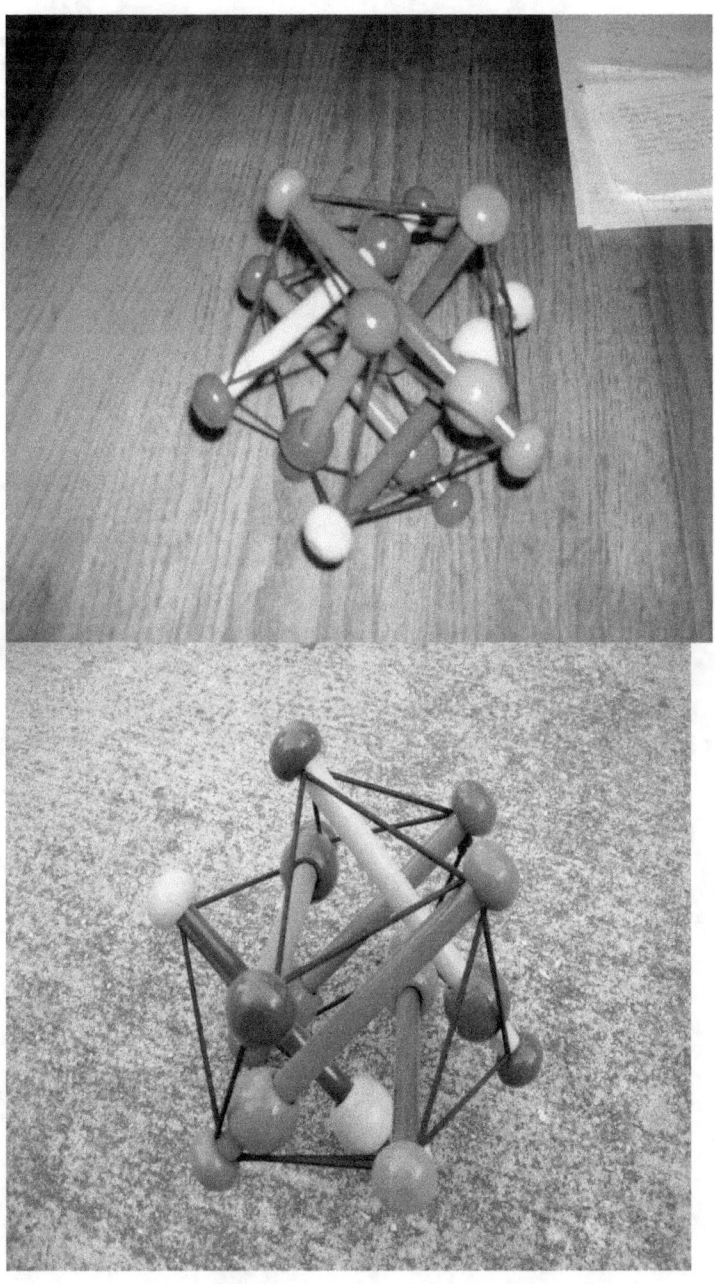

These are called *tensegrity* figures. The term was coined by Buckminster Fuller and describes a structure comprising "islands of compression in a sea of tension". Note that none of the dowels touch; they are held in place by the tension of the elastic bands.

One of the key features of a tensegrity structure is that changes in tension in one spot will have an effect on the entire structure and the effect will be within the bounds of the state of tension in the entire structure.

Consider that none of the bones in your body touch and all are set at angles to each other while in a sea of elastic connective substance. YOU are a tensegrity structure!

You are NOT a compressive structure, like a stone column. Yet this is how people tend to view themselves and their actions. Your knees don't compress; nor does your vertebrae. And there is no pressure on the bones in your feet.

Your bones work as "spacers", much like the dowels in the tensegrity structure. There is not a bone in your structure that is not surrounded by all sorts of networks devoted to the distribution and transformation of compression/tension.

This network of tension acts as a global "web" system and the changes in joint angles work like "routers" across the network. Your neural system would then act as a "web crawler" system building an index of repeated patterns. This connective network maintains a steady state of tension and fixed angular relationships so that the entire system only has to deal with notable changes in tensional states.

If you were not "pre-tensed", there would be no efficient or dependable means of starting movement or detecting changes because you would have no fixed and constant frame of reference with which to work. It would be like having a compass that never regularly indicated any direction – worse than useless.

This "pre-tension" is a key element in learning to move with ease instead of fighting your way through movement.

Some of your connective tissues are semi-elastic (pre-tension). Like the cartilage in your ears, they can be bent or distorted to a certain degree and will snap back to their original shape. The energy generated by the muscles and the bones act to apply the distorting pressure. So, changes in the angles of your joints deform the connective tissue and the tendency to restore shape becomes stored elastic energy.

It is much better to learn or practice a physical skill in terms of angular changes/modulation. For instance, if you are trying to learn how to do a handstand, nearly everyone will coach you by telling you to "throw" your legs up in the air and then train your muscles to arrest the momentum of your legs and consciously make efforts to tense the muscles that you *believe* to be the ones necessary for maintaining balance.

But more careful examination reveals that as your legs move, corresponding angular changes are occurring throughout the body. It is these angular changes that people struggle against when learning to "muscle" the technique. Now, alignment is alignment, whether you are inverted or standing upright. If you take for granted that your body aligns itself when you stand and walk, why would you think that you need to learn how to force yourself to align when you are inverted? There's no less tension in your cartilage and your bones don't fit less snugly just because your feet are over your head!

You can muscle your way into position, but you're only going to end up in the same alignment that your structure would go to anyway. Using your natural angular modulation is far more efficient – it burns far less energy.

Using/burning energy and releasing energy can be viewed here as different things. When you rely on angular modulation, you are storing and releasing energy (when you deform a joint angle, this change is an energetic state that releases energy when the angle returns to its beginning state). A simple shift in your angular relationship to the ground is enough to cause an energetic state to occur. Note that any shift in your gravitational relationship will involve global angular changes.

When you try to *force* an isolated angular change, as in trying to "use your abs" or "kick up fast" or "push hard with your arms", you recruit heavy muscular activation. This heavy recruitment burns lots of fuel to generate energy, which helps movement but also releases large amounts of heat.

Matching natural angular modulation to your gravitational alignment releases energy while burning minute amounts of fuel because your muscles act only to correct small linear deviations.

As I said earlier, your body is tensegral in nature, but unlike the tensegrity figure in the photos, you also have some "floating" pivots that give a limited degree of freedom to certain angular changes. One of these floating pivot systems is the deltoid and the other main floating pivot system is the pelvic structure. These two systems are interrelated, and changes in one will be reflected by changes in the other. This is vitally important to understand, especially if you play football or engage in some other activity that requires sudden, sharp changes in direction of travel.

These two systems *counter-rotate*; when the pelvis angles to the right, your shoulders will angle to the left and vice versa. This is why your arms will naturally have a tendency to cross in front of your pelvis. For example, in football, when you run down the field and suddenly cut to the right, your pelvis *should* angle sharply to the right while your right arm swings hard to your left. This should happen whether you start your pivot on your left foot **or** your right. This way, your mass/weight pivots at the pelvis and stress is distributed and transformed by the powerful hip structure. Problems like torn knee ligaments occur when the pivot takes place at the *knee*.

Remember, the body likes alignment; so when the pelvis starts angling out of alignment with the feet, a tremendous amount of energy is being generated and stored. Angling the shoulders in opposition of the pelvis conserves this energy in the massive hip structure whereas if the shoulders and pelvis angle in the same direction, this energy will be conserved in the much smaller knee structure.

Energy should be stored in the pelvic system and released through the limbs – NOT stored and released in the limbs alone.

The study of the importance of the pelvis/hip system (in energy transformation) forms the core teachings of yoga/Asian martial arts.

The basic relationship between the pelvis and shoulders (also called the lunar plexus and solar plexus, respectively) is explored in the positions such as the Warrior poses and their transitions. In karate, the front stance and the reverse punch are an exploration of the power of counter-rotation.

(Mr. Myagi was telling the truth when he told Daniel-san that the secret of Okinawan karate could be found in rotating that little drum back and forth (in The Karate Kid Part II); karate techniques are indeed a way to observe the workings of the universe).

For instance, when executing a reverse punch (right hand punching from a left leg-forward stance), the pelvis and shoulders move together to your left; but at the last second, the pelvis angles sharply to the right and this generates the extra energy people call "snap" in the punch.

Now let's look at the left downward block executed in a left front stance (left foot forward). Your left hand travels downward from your right shoulder to a point above your left knee. As your hand reaches its final destination to your left, your pelvis will angle sharply to your right. At the same time, your right hand will travel back and to your right to come to rest at your hip. As you do this, you will notice that your shoulders don't do much angling either way. AHA! The counter-rotation of the shoulders is replaced by your left arm traveling in a big line to your left while your right arm travels a short distance to your right. This trade-off works because it's about *conservation of energy* rather than your concept of arms and legs being separate "parts". In other words, it doesn't matter whether the energy is conserved by your "arms" or your "shoulders", energy is energy, and your arms can conserve as much energy as your shoulders because of their greater rotation.

Some of you may wonder about punches thrown where there is no counter-rotation at the end of the strike, like in a boxer's jab and/or cross. Well, there *is* counter-rotation; it's just done on the other side.

In the karate reverse punch, as the right hand reaches extension, the pelvis rotates sharply to the right so that pelvis and right arm move in opposite directions. In the boxer's right cross, the pelvis will rotate all the way to the left as the right arm extends (also to the left). The right arm and the pelvis travel in the same direction. But once the pelvis begins to angle to the left, the left hand (held high - to at least shoulder level) moves slightly forward *and to the right*. So the left hand (guarding the face) moves in opposition to the pelvic direction as the right hand fully extends.

Though there is no sharp directional change in pelvic motion, there is still conservation of angular energy through opposing arm activity.

If we look at the boxer's jab, we see the same functions at work, but without a full 90° pelvic rotation. The left hand extends (jabs) and the pelvis angles to the right. As the pelvis angles, the right hand (held high) and shoulder tighten towards the left, providing counter pressure against the pelvic action.

The reason that all this counter rotation is important is simple: remember what happens when the elbow extends away from the body and beyond the foot - you will automatically take a step to realign your structure as in the set up for the judo foot sweep. Your physiology demands that your center of mass/weight fall *between* the feet.

Now, you may wonder why you would *not* want your body weight to move out in the same direction as you punch. The reason is simple: once your center of mass/weight moves out of vertical alignment, your connective system makes *re-alignment* a priority; distributing and transferring force to a target takes a backseat to maintaining structural integrity. Also bear in mind that a big part of alignment AND energy transference is highly dependent upon friction and friction is a coefficient of weight. When you are moving out of alignment, there is less weight (pressure) on your feet and thus, less friction.

If you were to try to throw a sharp jab with your left while keeping your right hand extended out to your right, you would find that your pelvis and deep abdominal muscles won't activate forcefully.

From a defensive or counter-attacking perspective, knowing that these angular details are necessary in order for your opponent to transfer full power to you, you now know exactly what can be done to disrupt the process.

Counter-rotation keeps you center of mass/gravity between your feet.

The uniform and fixed structure of the human being is how a Zen archer can put an arrow into a bullseye and then split that same arrow with another, even while unable to see the target. With a heightened sensitivity honed by decades of practice, the archer knows that repeating the same angular changes in the body will produce identical results in the release of the arrow.

Further study reveals that the same angular changes done in a different context can produce *emergent* results. This is why, to your structure, a kettlebell swing, strand pulling, yoga poses and throwing a football are all the same thing, even though we think of them as different actions. The only differences are in the final expression; the generating processes are identical. *To know one thing deeply is to know the entire universe.*

When "springing" skills are coached (like in jumping sports or tumbling and gymnastics), much is spoken about the "blocking action" where you plant a limb at about a 45° angle and use this angle to generate upward velocity (sometimes this is called the penultimate step).

In reality, this is a method of angulation being used to direct and store energy. The angling makes use of elastic re-alignment (or stored elastic energy) to not only store elastic energy in the connective tissues, but the angle also extends the amount of *time* in which you store and release the energy. The point of this is to show you that in your mind, there is a "you" doing a bunch of different "things". In reality, it's all nothing but transformations of energy expressed through changes in the relationship between time and distance (seen as angular modulation).

In closing, the thing to remember is that piling on more and more trivia, factoids, techniques and second-hand knowledge is no substitute for true understanding. And the thing to understand is that *you are not some "thing" living in the universe*; **you ARE the universe**.